Vitamin D
and
Vitamin C

The Dynamic Duo for Optimal Health

By

John E. Ramirez

Author's Disclaimer

The contents of this book are intended for informational purposes only and should not be considered a substitute for professional medical, nutritional, or psychological advice, diagnosis, or treatment. The author is not a medical professional, and the information provided is based on personal research and experience.
Readers are encouraged to consult with qualified healthcare professionals for any specific health concerns, conditions, or dietary needs. Any actions or decisions made based on the information in this book are the sole responsibility of the reader.

By reading this book, the reader acknowledges and accepts these disclaimers. It is advised to consult a qualified healthcare professional for any medical, nutritional, or psychological concerns.

TABLE OF CONTENTS

INTRODUCTION

Few substances are as important as vitamins in the rich tapestry of human health. These chemical components, which are often overlooked in our fast-paced modern lifestyles, are the unsung heroes who silently orchestrate a symphony of critical processes within our bodies. Among these extraordinary vitamins, two stand out as standouts: vitamin D and vitamin C. We will discover the intricate roles, profound impacts, and interesting interplay of these two exceptional nutrients as we explore through the pages of this book.

Vitamin D, also known as the "sunshine vitamin," takes us into the enthralling world of sunlight and its significant impact on our health. In the chapters of this book, we'll delve into the complexities of bone health, immune system fortification, and even mood control that are carefully sewn into the fabric of this multipurpose vitamin.

Then we go on to Vitamin C, the strong antioxidant that conjures up visions of brilliant citrus fruits and the tangy blast of flavor that comes with every bite.

However, its influence extends far beyond taste. Its chemical structure contains the ability to protect our cells from the ravages of oxidative stress, boost the creation of collagen, which gives our skin and bones strength, and strengthen our immune defenses against the onslaught of contemporary life.

We will go through these pages from the historical discoveries that brought these vitamins to light to the cutting-edge research that is now unraveling their mysteries. We'll look at how these vitamins interact with our bodies, how they interact with each system, each cell, and each delicate balance that keeps us healthy.

We ask you to join us on this journey of knowledge and discovery as we explore the intriguing worlds of Vitamin D and Vitamin C.

CHAPTER ONE: INTRODUCTION TO VITAMINS

What Exactly Are Vitamins?

Vitamins are chemical substances that are necessary for several physiological functions in the human body. They are necessary at modest levels for proper functioning, growth, and overall health maintenance. While the body can synthesize some vitamins, many must be received from diet or supplements because the body's production is frequently insufficient to meet the body's demands.

Vitamins are divided into two. They are water-soluble vitamins and fat-soluble vitamins.

- Water-Soluble Vitamins: Vitamin C and the B-complex vitamins (B1, B2, B3, B6, B9, and B12) are examples of water-soluble vitamins. These vitamins are water-soluble and are not significantly stored in the body. They are easily absorbed from the gastrointestinal system and, if ingested in excess, are expelled in the urine. Because of their water solubility, they must be ingested on a regular basis as part of a well-balanced diet.

- Fat-Soluble Vitamins: Examples of Fat-Soluble Vitamins are Vitamins A, D, E, and K. These vitamins are fat-soluble and are absorbed in conjunction with dietary lipids. Unlike water-soluble vitamins, fat-soluble vitamins can be stored for longer periods of time in the body's fat cells and liver, lowering the need for daily ingestion. Excessive use of fat-soluble vitamins, on the other hand, might cause toxicity because they are not easily eliminated.

These vitamins help in energy metabolism, neurological function, red blood cell creation, and DNA synthesis, among other things. Vitamin C functions as an antioxidant, promoting immunological function, collagen formation, and wound healing. Each vitamin has a specific purpose and contributes to overall health. Any vitamin deficiency can result in a variety of health problems and diseases. To guarantee an appropriate intake of vitamins, it is critical to have a balanced diet rich in fruits, vegetables, whole grains, and lean proteins. Dietary supplements may be required in some circumstances to achieve vitamin requirements, particularly in individuals with specific dietary limitations or medical problems.

Consultation with a healthcare practitioner or certified dietitian can assist in determining the proper vitamin consumption based on individual needs and health goals. Excessive intake of certain vitamins can also be dangerous; thus, it is critical to follow established dietary restrictions and avoid mega doses of vitamins without professional assistance.

Vitamins' Importance in Human Health

Vitamins are necessary micronutrients that play an important role in overall health and well-being. They are needed in modest amounts, but their absence or shortage can cause a variety of health concerns. Vitamins have a role in a variety of physiological processes in the body, and their significance in human health cannot be emphasized. Here are some significant areas where vitamins are important:

1. Energy Production and Metabolism: Vitamins, namely B-complex vitamins (B1, B2, B3, B5, B6, B7, B9, and B12), are required for the conversion of food into energy. They work as coenzymes in metabolic reactions, assisting the body in breaking

down carbs, lipids, and proteins to provide energy that powers biological operations.

2. Cell Development and Repair: Vitamins are necessary for cell development, replication, and repair. They promote DNA synthesis, cell division, and overall cellular health, ensuring that the body's tissues and organs work properly.

3. Immune System Function: Certain vitamins, such as vitamin C and vitamin D, play critical roles in immune system support. Vitamin C is well-known for its antioxidant capabilities, which aid in the protection of immune cells against oxidative damage. Vitamin D participates in immune cell regulation and improves the body's ability to fight infections.

4. Antioxidant Defense: Vitamin C, Vitamin E, and beta-carotene act as antioxidants that scavenge dangerous free radicals that can damage cells and contribute to chronic diseases such as cancer, cardiovascular disease, and aging.

5. Bone Health and Mineralization: Vitamin D is essential for calcium absorption in the intestines and for normal bone health. It maintains blood calcium and phosphorus levels, facilitating bone

mineralization and preventing disorders such as osteoporosis.

6. Blood Clotting and Wound Healing: Vitamin K is required for blood clotting as well as wound healing. It aids in the synthesis of proteins involved in the creation of blood clots and bone metabolism.

7. Neurological Function: B vitamins, particularly B6, B9 (folate), and B12, are required for normal neurological function. They help to maintain neuron health, neurotransmitter production, and cognitive functions.

8. Skin Health and Collagen Production: Vitamin C is essential for collagen production, a protein that gives skin, joints, and blood vessels structure. It supports skin health, wound healing, and helps connective tissue integrity.

9. Vision and Eye Health: Vitamin A is vital for keeping good vision since it supports retinal health and low-light and color vision.

10. Hormone Regulation: Vitamins have a role in the manufacture and regulation of hormones, which are essential for many biological activities such as metabolism, growth, and reproduction.

11.   Formation of Red Blood Cells: Vitamin B12 and folate are required for the formation of red blood cells, which transport oxygen throughout the body.

It's crucial to remember that while vitamins are necessary for good health, more isn't always better. Certain vitamin deficits and excesses can both be harmful to one's health. A balanced diet rich in nutrient-dense foods is essential for ensuring optimal vitamin consumption. If you suspect a deficiency or have specific health problems, it is best to speak with a healthcare expert or certified dietitian.

Classification of Vitamin

Vitamins are chemical substances that are required by the body for a variety of physiological activities. Based on their solubility in water and fat, they are divided into two major groups:

1. Vitamins that are soluble in water: Water-soluble vitamins dissolve in water and are not extensively stored in the body. They must be consumed on a regular basis because excess amounts are expelled rather than stored. Among the water-soluble vitamins are:

a. Vitamin C (Ascorbic Acid): Vitamin C is well-known for its antioxidant effects, and it helps the immune system, collagen formation, and wound healing. It also improves iron absorption and promotes healthy skin.

b. B1 (Thiamine): Thiamine is required for the conversion of carbohydrates into energy, as well as for nerve function and general metabolism.

c. B2 (Riboflavin): Riboflavin is involved in energy synthesis, cellular development, and lipid, drug, and steroid metabolism.

d. B3 (Niacin): Niacin helps with energy generation, DNA repair, and skin and nerve health.

e. Pantothenic acid (B5): Pantothenic acid is a coenzyme. A component that is essential for several metabolic processes, including energy production and fatty acid synthesis.

f. Pyridoxine (B6) is required for protein metabolism, neurotransmitter production, and immune system function.

g. B7 (Biotin): Biotin is required for healthy skin, hair, and nails and is involved in carbohydrates, fat, and protein metabolism.

h. B9 (Folate or Folic Acid): Folate is required for DNA synthesis, cell division, and red blood cell development. It is especially critical during pregnancy to avoid neural tube abnormalities.

i. B12 (Cobalamin): Vitamin B12 is required for the development of red blood cells, neuron function, DNA synthesis, and general metabolism.

2. Fat-Soluble Vitamins: Fat-soluble vitamins dissolve in fat and are stored in the fatty tissues and liver of the body. Excessive consumption of fat-soluble vitamins might induce toxicity since they can be stored. Among the fat-soluble vitamins are:

a. Retinol (Vitamin A): Retinol is essential for vision, immunological function, skin health, and cell differentiation. It is also necessary for the health of the eyes, skin, and mucous membranes.

b. Vitamin D(Calciferol): Calcium and phosphorus absorption, bone health, immune system regulation, and overall well-being all rely on vitamin D (calciferol). It is also known as the "sunshine vitamin" since it may be synthesized by the skin when exposed to sunlight.

c. Vitamin E (Tocopherol): As an antioxidant, vitamin E protects cells from oxidative damage. It helps to maintain healthy skin and immunological function.

d. Vitamin K (Phylloquinone, Menadione): Vitamin K is required for the manufacture of clotting components, which is required for blood coagulation. It is also beneficial to bone health and may have anti-inflammatory qualities.

It is critical to maintain good health by balancing the intake of both water-soluble and fat-soluble vitamins. A diversified and well-rounded diet rich in nutrient-dense foods is the best strategy to ensure optimal vitamin intake.

CHAPTER TWO: VITAMIN D THE SUNSHINE VITAMIN

Overview of Vitamin D

Vitamin D is a fat-soluble vitamin that is required for several biological processes. It aids the body's absorption of calcium and phosphorus from food, both of which are required for the development and maintenance of strong bones and teeth. Furthermore, vitamin D is essential for immune system regulation, cell growth and communication, and inflammation reduction.

There are two forms of Vitamin D: Vitamin D2 (ergocalciferol) and Vitamin D3 (cholecalciferol). Vitamin D2 is derived mostly from plants, but vitamin D3 is created when the skin is exposed to sunshine and can also be obtained from certain animal-based meals.

For most people, exposure to sunlight is their principal source of vitamin D. When the sun's ultraviolet-B (UVB) rays strike the skin, a chemical reaction occurs that converts a molecule called 7-dehydrocholesterol into vitamin D3. Geographic location, season, time of day, cloud cover, skin pigmentation, and sunscreen use, on the other hand, can all influence vitamin D production in the skin.

Fatty fish such as salmon and mackerel, cod liver oil, fortified dairy products, fortified cereals, and egg yolks are all good sources of vitamin D. Vitamin D insufficiency is a frequent ailment around the world, with certain groups being especially vulnerable. Individuals with minimal sun exposure, such as those who are homebound or reside in higher latitudes, persons with darker skin pigmentation, older adults, people who wear clothing that covers most of their skin, and those with disorders that hinder fat absorption in the intestines, are among those who are at risk.

Symptoms of vitamin D insufficiency can range from weariness to muscle weakness to bone discomfort, as well as recurrent infections, depression, and delayed wound healing.

Supplementation is frequently suggested to prevent and cure vitamin D insufficiency. The recommended dietary allowance (RDA) for vitamin D varies according to age, gender, and stage of life. The RDA for adults is 600 to 800 international units (IU) per day. Higher doses, on the other hand, may be given by healthcare professionals for those with certain diseases or risk factors.

It is vital to highlight that excessive vitamin D use might be dangerous. This can occur because of excessive supplementation or intake of vitamin D-fortified foods. Nausea, vomiting, poor appetite, constipation, weakness, and kidney issues are all symptoms of vitamin D intoxication.

Finally, vitamin D is necessary for bone health, immunological function, cell growth, and communication. Adequate sun exposure, combined with a well-balanced diet and maybe supplementation, is essential for maintaining adequate vitamin D levels and avoiding insufficiency. It is, nevertheless, critical to speak with a healthcare practitioner to decide the optimum dose of vitamin D for your unique needs.

Sources of Vitamin D

Vitamin D is an unusual vitamin in that it may be generated by the body when exposed to sunshine. It is also available via food sources and supplements. The following are the key sources of vitamin D:

1. Exposure to sunlight: Sunlight is the greatest and most important natural source of vitamin D. When the skin is exposed to UVB rays from the sun, a type of cholesterol in the skin is changed into a precursor of vitamin D, which is subsequently processed into its active form by the liver and kidneys. The amount of vitamin D produced is affected by factors such as skin color, geographic location, time of day, and skin exposure. While sunshine is a great source of vitamin D, it's crucial to balance it with skin cancer preventive methods like sunscreen and protective clothes.

2. Dietary Sources: While the body may generate vitamin D from sunlight, dietary sources are also necessary for maintaining appropriate levels, especially when solar exposure is limited. Here are some vitamin D-rich foods:

    a. Fatty Fish: Fatty fish is a good natural source of vitamin D. They are high in vitamin D and omega-3 fatty acids, both of which are good for your heart and brain. Examples of vitamin D-rich fatty fish include Salmon, Mackerel, Sardines, Trout, Tuna, Herring.

b. Cod Liver Oil: Cod liver oil is taken from the liver of cod fish and is a good source of vitamin D and vitamin A. It is a dietary supplement that contains a high concentration of these vitamins.

c. Egg Yolks: Egg yolks contain trace quantities of vitamin D. The amount varies depending on the nutrition of the hens which laid the eggs. Eggs are a flexible food that may be used in a variety of cuisines to increase vitamin D intake.

d. Mushrooms: Some species of mushrooms naturally contain trace quantities of vitamin D, particularly when grown in direct sunshine. In addition, certain mushroom varieties are treated with ultraviolet light to boost their vitamin D content.

e. Beef Liver: Beef liver contains a variety of minerals, including vitamin D. It also contains iron, vitamin A, and other vitamins and minerals.

f. Cheese: Some cheeses, such as cheddar and Swiss, contain trace quantities of vitamin D. Cheese can be eaten as a snack or added to meals.

g. Tofu: Some kinds of tofu are fortified with vitamin D, making it a viable alternative for vegetarian or vegan diets.

h. Pork: Pork products, such as pork chops and loin, include a considerable quantity of vitamin D.

3. Fortified Foods: Fortified foods are goods that have certain nutrients added to them to increase their nutritional worth. Fortification is a technique that is often used to alleviate nutrient shortages and increase the overall nutritious content of meals. Here are some vitamin D-fortified foods that are commonly consumed:

a. Fortified Milk and Dairy Products: Cow's milk and dairy products are frequently supplemented with vitamin D to assist people fulfill their daily requirements. This contains items such as:

- Regular Milk

- Milk with a lower fat content

- Skimmed Milk

- Yogurt

- Cheese

b. Plant-Based Milk Substitutes: Many plant-based milk alternatives, such as almond milk, soy milk, and oat milk, are vitamin D fortified, making them a viable option for people who are lactose intolerant or follow a vegan diet.

c. Breakfast Cereals: Some breakfast cereals, particularly those aimed at delivering critical nutrients, are vitamin D fortified. These cereals might be a quick and easy method to increase your vitamin D consumption in the morning.

d. Orange Juice: Certain kinds of orange juice are enriched with vitamin D, providing a tasty and refreshing method to get this key ingredient.

e. Breads & Baked products: Some breads, rolls, and other baked products may be vitamin D fortified, adding to your daily dose.

f. Margarines and Spreads: Certain margarines and spreads are fortified with vitamin D, making them an easy and varied method to include this component in your diet.

g. Cereal Bars and Snack Bars: Some cereal bars and snack bars, like morning cereals, may contain additional vitamin D to provide a convenient and portable source of nutrition.

Fortified foods can be especially advantageous for people who get a little sun, as well as those who have dietary limitations or preferences that make it difficult to get enough vitamin D from natural sources. It is critical to study labels when selecting fortified foods to establish the amount of vitamin D added and to ensure that the product fits into your entire dietary plan.

4. Supplements: Vitamin D pills are a simple way to guarantee that you're getting enough of this crucial nutrient, especially if you don't receive enough sun exposure or have trouble getting enough vitamin D from dietary sources. Supplements can be especially advantageous for people who have certain health concerns, live in areas with minimal sunlight, or follow specific eating habits. What you should know about vitamin D pills is as follows:

   a. Types of Vitamin D Supplements: The types of vitamin D supplements are:

   - Ergocalciferol (Vitamin D2): This form is obtained from plants and is often used in supplements. It is efficient at increasing vitamin D levels in the blood.

- Cholecalciferol (Vitamin D3): When the skin is exposed to sunshine, vitamin D3 (cholecalciferol) is created from cholesterol. Some animal-based foods contain it as well. Supplements containing vitamin D3 are thought to be more effective at increasing and maintaining vitamin D levels in the body.

b. Who Might Benefit from Supplements: The following are people who might benefit from supplements:

- People who get little sun exposure, such as those who live in cold climates or spend most of their time indoors.

- Melanin in the skin lowers the skin's ability to synthesize vitamin D in reaction to sunshine, hence people with darker skin are at a disadvantage.

- Senior citizens, as the skin's ability to produce vitamin D diminishes with age.

- People who conceal their skin for religious or cultural reasons.

- Individuals suffering from medical problems that impair vitamin D absorption or metabolism.

c. Suggested Dosages: The suggested amount of vitamin D supplements varies depending on age, health status, and individual demands. To establish the optimum dosage for your case, consult with a healthcare expert.

d. Excessive Intake Should Be Avoided: While vitamin D is necessary for health, too much of it can cause vitamin D toxicity, also known as hypervitaminosis D. This can cause high blood calcium levels, which can cause symptoms such as nausea, vomiting, weakness, and kidney difficulties. Before taking high-dose supplements, it's critical to stick to the suggested amounts and consult with a healthcare practitioner.

e. Supplement Selection: When choosing a Vitamin D supplement, the following should be considered:

- Vitamin D3 tablets are more effective at increasing and maintaining vitamin D levels.

- Look for items that have undergone third-party testing for content quality and accuracy.

- Choose a dosage that corresponds to your unique needs and the advice of your healthcare practitioner.

f. Interaction with Other Drugs: Some drugs and medical conditions can interact with vitamin D supplements. Consult your healthcare practitioner if you're taking other medications or have underlying health concerns.

Remember that while supplements can be a beneficial tool, they should complement a balanced diet and a healthy lifestyle. It's important to see a healthcare practitioner before starting any supplements plan to confirm that it's acceptable for your unique demands and health situation.

Functions of Vitamin D

Vitamin D is a versatile nutrient with a wide range of effects throughout the body. It plays a key part in sustaining general health, and its functions extend beyond merely bone health. Here are some of the important functions of vitamin D:

1. Calcium and Phosphorus Absorption: Vitamin D is important for the absorption of calcium and phosphorus in the intestines. It helps manage the amounts of these minerals in the blood, encouraging their uptake from the digestive system into the bloodstream. Adequate calcium and phosphorus levels are critical for keeping bones and teeth strong.
2. Bone Health: One of the most well-known effects of Vitamin D is its role in bone health. Vitamin D works together with calcium to ensure that bones are calcified effectively. It increases the deposition of calcium and phosphorus into the bone matrix, making bones robust and resilient.
3. Bone Growth and Remodeling: Vitamin D is needed for bone growth and remodeling, which entails the ongoing breakdown and synthesis of bone structure. It helps regulate the balance between bone resorption (breakdown) and bone production, which is vital for preserving bone density and structure.
4. Immune System Regulation: Vitamin D plays a role in modifying the immune system. It has been demonstrated to alter the function of immune cells,

such as macrophages and T cells, helping the body fight off infections and respond to inflammation.

5. Anti-Inflammatory Effects: Vitamin D possesses anti-inflammatory qualities that can help manage the body's inflammatory response. Adequate vitamin D levels may help minimize the risk of chronic inflammatory diseases.

6. Cell Growth and Differentiation: Vitamin D is involved in controlling cell growth and differentiation. It helps control how cells grow, mature, and specialize, which is vital for maintaining healthy tissues and preventing the growth of malignant cells.

7. Hormone Regulation: Vitamin D operates as a hormone by attaching to specific receptors on cells throughout the body. These receptors are located in different tissues, including the brain, heart, and immune system, showing the widespread influence of vitamin D on various physiological processes.

8. Nervous System Health: Vitamin D is known to play a role in neurological health and cognitive performance. It may support nerve growth and transmission, contributing to general brain health.

9. Cardiovascular Health: Some evidence suggests that vitamin D may have a preventive impact on cardiovascular health. Adequate vitamin D levels are related to a lower risk of certain cardiovascular diseases.

10. Mood Regulation: Vitamin D has been connected to mood regulation and mental wellness. Low vitamin D levels have been related to an increased risk of mood disorders like depression.

11. Gene Expression: Vitamin D can alter gene expression by interacting with certain genes involved in distinct cellular processes. This allows vitamin D to affect a wide range of biological functions.

Maintaining optimum vitamin D levels is critical for supporting these functions and general health. While the most well-known job of vitamin D is its support for bone health, its influence extends to many other elements of the body's functioning. Ensuring appropriate vitamin D intake through solar exposure, food sources, and supplementation (if necessary) can assist support these vital functions.

Vitamin D deficiency happens when the body doesn't obtain enough of this crucial nutrient to maintain optimal health. It can lead to a range of health concerns due to the vital function vitamin D plays in different physiological processes. Here are some of the health effects of vitamin D deficiency:

1. Bone Health Issues: One of the most well-known implications of vitamin D insufficiency is decreased bone health. Without sufficient vitamin D, the body struggles to absorb enough calcium and phosphorus, resulting in weaker bones. In youngsters, severe deficiency can induce rickets, a disorder characterized by soft and weak bones. In adults, vitamin D insufficiency can develop into osteomalacia, which leads to bone discomfort, muscle weakness, and an increased risk of fractures.

2. Weakened Immune Function: Vitamin D plays a critical function in immune system modulation. A deficit can decrease the immune response, rendering the body more prone to infections, including respiratory tract infections.

3. Increased Risk of Chronic Diseases: There is growing evidence associating vitamin D deficiency with an increased risk of chronic diseases. Low vitamin D levels have been connected with illnesses such as cardiovascular disease, diabetes, hypertension, autoimmune disorders, and certain forms of cancer.

While the association between deficiency and various disorders is complex and not fully understood, keeping enough vitamin D levels is considered vital for overall health.

4. Muscular Weakness and Pain: Vitamin D insufficiency has been linked to muscular weakness and pain. Adequate vitamin D levels are necessary for muscle function, and a lack of it can contribute to muscle weakness, cramping, and widespread discomfort.

5. Increased Fall Risk in Older Persons: Older persons with vitamin D insufficiency are at a higher risk of falls and fractures due to reduced bone health and muscle strength. Maintaining appropriate vitamin D levels may help lower the incidence of falls and related injuries.

6. Mood Disorders: Some research suggests a potential link between low vitamin D levels and mood disorders such as depression and seasonal affective disorder (SAD). While the exact relationship is complex and not entirely understood, vitamin D's role in brain health and neurotransmitter control may contribute to these relationships.

7. Impaired Wound Healing: Adequate vitamin D is crucial for wound healing and tissue repair. Vitamin D deficiency can slow down the healing process and hinder the body's capacity to recover from injuries and procedures.

8. Pregnancy Complications: Pregnant women with vitamin D deficiency may be at a higher risk of complications such as gestational diabetes, preeclampsia, and poor fetal development. Sufficient vitamin D is vital for the health of both the mother and the developing fetus.

Risk Factors for Deficiency

Certain factors can increase the risk of vitamin D deficiency, including limited sun exposure, living at higher latitudes, having darker skin, older age, obesity, certain medical conditions that affect vitamin D absorption, and following a strict vegan or vegetarian diet.

To maintain overall health and well-being, it is important to prevent the risk of vitamin D deficiency. If you suspect a deficiency or have risk factors, it's advisable to consult a healthcare professional. They can assess your vitamin D levels through blood tests and provide guidance on appropriate sun exposure, dietary changes, and supplementation if necessary.

Rickets and Osteomalacia

Rickets and osteomalacia are two related medical conditions that result from a deficiency of vitamin D, calcium, or phosphorus. These conditions primarily affect bone health and can lead to weakened bones and other health problems. Here's an overview of rickets and osteomalacia:

1. Rickets: Rickets is a condition that primarily affects children during their growing years when bones are still developing and mineralizing. It is characterized by the inadequate mineralization of bone tissue, leading to soft and weakened bones. Rickets most commonly occur due to a deficiency of vitamin D, calcium, or phosphorus. Vitamin D deficiency is a major cause of rickets because vitamin D plays a crucial role in the absorption of calcium and phosphorus, which are essential for building strong bones.

   Symptoms of rickets can include:

   - Bowing of the legs or knock-knees

- The curvature of the spine (scoliosis)

- Delayed growth and development

- Muscle weakness

- Dental problems

- Pain and tenderness in bones

- Fractures that occur easily

Rickets can have long-lasting effects on bone development and overall health if not treated promptly. It's important to address the underlying deficiency and provide appropriate treatment to prevent complications.

2. Osteomalacia: Osteomalacia is a condition that primarily affects adults. It is characterized by the softening of bones due to inadequate mineralization. Like rickets, osteomalacia can result from a deficiency of vitamin D, calcium, or phosphorus. In osteomalacia, the bones are already formed but are not properly mineralized, leading to weakness, pain, and an increased risk of fractures.

Symptoms of osteomalacia can include:

- Bone pain, often in the lower back, hips, and legs

- Muscle weakness

- Fractures with minimal trauma
- Difficulty walking or moving

Osteomalacia is often caused by chronic vitamin D deficiency or conditions that affect vitamin D metabolism, such as kidney disorders that impair vitamin D activation. It's important to address the underlying cause of osteomalacia and provide treatment to improve bone health and alleviate symptoms.

Prevention and Treatment

Both rickets and osteomalacia are preventable and treatable conditions. Adequate intake of vitamin D, calcium, and phosphorus through diet, sunlight exposure, and supplementation (under medical supervision) is essential. For individuals with diagnosed deficiencies, healthcare professionals may recommend appropriate supplements and dietary changes.

If you suspect that you or someone you know may have symptoms of rickets or osteomalacia, it's important to consult a healthcare provider. A proper diagnosis and treatment plan can help prevent further complications and promote optimal bone health.

Increase Risk of Chronic Disease

Research suggests that vitamin D deficiency may be related to an increase in the risk of various chronic diseases. While the exact mechanisms are still being studied, there is growing evidence that maintaining adequate vitamin D levels is important for overall health and disease prevention. Here are some of the chronic diseases that have been linked to vitamin D deficiency:

1. Cardiovascular Disease: Some studies have suggested a potential link between low vitamin D levels and an increased risk of cardiovascular disease. Vitamin D may play a role in regulating blood pressure, reducing inflammation, improving endothelial function, and supporting overall heart health.
2. Type 2 Diabetes: Vitamin D deficiency has been associated with insulin resistance and impaired glucose metabolism, which are risk factors for type 2 diabetes. Adequate vitamin D levels may help improve insulin sensitivity and reduce the risk of developing diabetes.
3. Cancer: There is ongoing research into the relationship between vitamin D and cancer risk. Some studies have shown associations between low vitamin D levels and an increased risk of certain

types of cancer, including breast, prostate, and colorectal cancers. Vitamin D's role in cell differentiation, immune regulation, and inflammation may contribute to its potential protective effects against cancer.

4. Autoimmune Diseases: Vitamin D deficiency has been linked to various autoimmune diseases, such as multiple sclerosis, rheumatoid arthritis, and systemic lupus erythematosus. Vitamin D's immunomodulatory properties may play a role in regulating immune responses and reducing the risk of autoimmune disorders.

5. Respiratory Infections: Adequate vitamin D levels may help support respiratory health and reduce the risk of respiratory infections. Vitamin D is believed to play a role in enhancing the body's defense mechanisms against infections and reducing inflammation in the respiratory tract.

6. Neurological Disorders: Some studies have suggested a potential association between vitamin D deficiency and neurological disorders such as Alzheimer's disease, Parkinson's disease, and cognitive decline. Vitamin D's role in neuronal function,

neuroprotection, and anti-inflammatory actions may contribute to its impact on brain health.

7. Mood Disorders: Studies have shown that low vitamin D levels can have an adverse increase in the risk of mood disorders such as depression. Vitamin D may play a role in serotonin synthesis and regulation, which can affect mood.

8. Bone Health (Osteoporosis): While the direct link between vitamin D deficiency and osteoporosis is well-established, osteoporosis is also considered a chronic disease with long-term implications. Vitamin D deficiency can lead to weakened bones and an increased risk of fractures, especially in older adults.

It's important to note that while these associations are being explored, the relationship between vitamin D deficiency and these chronic diseases is complex and multifactorial. Maintaining adequate vitamin D levels is just one aspect of a healthy lifestyle that includes a balanced diet, regular physical activity, and other factors that contribute to disease prevention. If you have concerns about your vitamin D levels or chronic disease risk, it's advisable to consult a healthcare professional for personalized guidance and recommendations.

Recommended Dietary Allowances (RDAs) For Vitamin D

The Recommended Dietary Allowances (RDAs) for vitamin D can vary based on age, gender, life stage, and individual factors. RDAs represent the average daily intake of a nutrient that is considered sufficient to meet the needs of most healthy individuals. Keep in mind that these recommendations are general guidelines, and individual needs may vary. The RDAs for vitamin D are:

- Infants (0-12 months): 400 international units (IU) per day (10 micrograms)

- Children (1-18 years): 600 IU per day (15 mcg)

- Adults (19-70 years): 600 IU per day (15 micrograms)

- Adults (71 years and older): 800 IU per day (20 micrograms)

- Pregnant and Lactating Women: 600 IU per day (15 mcg)

It's crucial to note that these RDAs are predicated on the assumption of low sun exposure, as sunshine is a substantial source of vitamin D production in the skin.

People who have limited sun exposure, reside at higher latitudes, have darker skin, or have certain medical disorders that impact vitamin D absorption may require increased vitamin D intake.

Additionally, individual demands can differ based on factors such as age, health status, pregnancy, breastfeeding, and overall dietary choices. Consulting with a healthcare practitioner can assist evaluate your unique vitamin D needs and whether supplementation is essential to achieve optimal levels.

If contemplating supplementing, it's crucial to find a recognized product and follow healthcare practitioner instructions to avoid excessive ingestion.

Controversies and Current Research on Vitamin D

Vitamin D is a topic of continuous research, and while it is a crucial nutrient with well-established effects, there are various areas of debate and current exploration. Here are some important disputes and current research areas connected to vitamin D:

1. Optimal Vitamin D Levels

Determining appropriate vitamin D levels is a topic of continuous research and controversy, as different health organizations and academics may have somewhat varying recommendations. The appropriate level of vitamin D in the blood varies depending on various factors, including age, health state, geographic region, and individual demands. Here are some general principles and recommendations for good vitamin D levels:

a. Measurement Units: Vitamin D levels are commonly measured in nanograms per milliliter (ng/mL) or nanomoles per liter (nmol/L). To convert between the two units, you can use the following approximate conversion: 1 ng/mL = 2.5 nmol/L.

b. Reference Ranges: Varying organizations and experts may have slightly varying reference ranges for vitamin D levels. However, the following ranges are typically referenced:

- Deficiency: Below 20 ng/mL (50 nmol/L)

- Insufficiency: 20-29 ng/mL (50-74 nmol/L)

- Adequate: 30-50 ng/mL (75-125 nmol/L)

- Optimal: Some experts indicate that optimal levels are in the range of 40-60 ng/mL (100-150 nmol/L) or somewhat higher.

c. Bone Health and Deficiency Prevention: To prevent disorders like rickets and osteomalacia, a vitamin D level of at least 20 ng/mL (50 nmol/L) is commonly suggested. This amount helps maintain optimal calcium absorption and bone health.

d. Extra Benefits and Chronic Disease Prevention: Some experts indicate that ideal vitamin D levels might be higher (about 40-60 ng/mL or 100-150 nmol/L) to potentially get extra health benefits, such as reducing the risk of chronic diseases like cardiovascular disease, diabetes, and some malignancies. However, these higher levels are still being examined, and definitive guidelines have not been consistently established.

e. Individual Variation: Optimal vitamin D levels can vary based on individual circumstances. Age, skin color, sun exposure, genetics, health issues, and lifestyle choices all play a role in defining what constitutes an appropriate amount for a specific person.

f. Clinical Assessment: It's crucial to note that identifying ideal levels is not a one-size-fits-all method. Healthcare specialists can examine your health condition, risk factors, and specific needs to help guide recommendations for vitamin D supplementation and maintaining optimal levels.

g. Consulting a Healthcare Professional: If you're concerned about your vitamin D levels, it's suggested to visit a healthcare expert. They can arrange blood tests to measure your vitamin D levels and make specific suggestions based on your health state and needs.

Remember that while aiming for adequate vitamin D levels is important, excessive vitamin D intake can lead to toxicity, which can have detrimental health implications. It's vital to achieve a balance between getting appropriate levels and avoiding excessive supplementation. Consulting a healthcare expert is essential to ensure that your vitamin D intake fits your needs and health goals.

2. Sun Exposure vs. Skin Cancer Risk

Sun exposure is a natural source of vitamin D production in the body, but it also carries the danger of skin damage and skin cancer, mostly owing to the harmful ultraviolet (UV) radiation from the sun. Balancing the benefits of sun exposure for vitamin D generation with the potential hazards of skin cancer is a vital factor. Here's how to strike a balance:

a. Vitamin D Synthesis: When your skin is exposed to UVB rays from the sun, a cholesterol component in your skin is transformed into vitamin D. This natural process is vital for maintaining enough vitamin D levels, which are important for bone health, immunological function, and overall well-being.

b. Skin Cancer Risk: Prolonged and unprotected exposure to UV radiation raises the risk of skin damage and skin cancer, including melanoma (the worst type of skin cancer), basal cell carcinoma, and squamous cell carcinoma.

c. Guidelines for Safe Sun Exposure: Follow these guidelines to optimize the advantages of sun exposure while limiting the danger of skin cancer:

- Brief Exposures: Short amounts of sun exposure (approximately 10-15 minutes) a few times per week, particularly during the noon sun, can help increase vitamin D synthesis without greatly raising the risk of skin cancer.

- Uncovered Skin: To increase vitamin D production during short exposure times, expose a greater area of skin, such as your arms, legs, back, or face.

- No Sunscreen: Avoid using sunscreen during the brief exposure period since it can impede the UVB rays required for vitamin D production.

d. Sun Protection Measures: To lower the risk of skin cancer when participating in outdoor activities, use the sun protection measures listed below:

- Apply Sunscreen: When spending long periods of time outside, especially during peak sun hours (10 a.m. to 4 p.m.), use a broad-spectrum sunscreen with at least SPF 30. Apply again every two hours, as well as after swimming or sweating.

- Clothing for Protection: To protect your skin from direct sun exposure, wear protective gear such as wide-brimmed hats, sunglasses, long-sleeved shirts, and slacks.

- Seek Shade: When feasible, seek shade, especially during peak sun hours when UV radiation is highest.

- Avoid using tanning beds: Tanning beds emit UV radiation and raise the risk of skin cancer; thus, they should be avoided at all costs.

e. Vitamin D Supplements: If receiving enough sun exposure is difficult owing to variables such as geographic location, lifestyle, or skin type, vitamin D supplements can be a safer option for maintaining optimal vitamin D levels without excessive sun exposure.

f. Consult a Medical Professional: Consult a healthcare expert if you are concerned about your vitamin D levels or the balance between sun exposure and skin cancer risk. They can make tailored recommendations based on your specific state of health, risk factors, and lifestyle.

While exposure to sunlight is necessary for vitamin D production, preserving your skin from damaging UV radiation and lowering your risk of skin cancer should be your focus. Maintaining optimal vitamin D levels through supplementation and food sources while encouraging general health and well-being is critical.

Immune Function and Vitamin D

Vitamin D is recognized to have an important part in immune system modulation, which is the body's defense mechanism against infections, illnesses, and foreign invaders. The relationship between vitamin D and immunological function is intricate and complicated. Here's how vitamin D affects immunological responses and how it affects overall immune health:

1. Immune Cell Regulation: Vitamin D has been demonstrated to affect the function of immune cells such as T cells, B cells, and macrophages. It can aid in the regulation of immune system components that are necessary for detecting and neutralizing dangerous microorganisms.
2. Strengthening Antimicrobial Defenses: Vitamin D stimulates the development of antimicrobial peptides, which are proteins with inherent antibiotic capabilities. These peptides aid the body's defense

against infections by damaging bacterial and viral cell membranes.

3. Anti-Inflammatory Characteristics: Vitamin D has anti-inflammatory characteristics that assist control the immunological response in the body. It can aid in the regulation of excessive inflammation, which is frequent in immune-related disorders.

4. Autoimmune Conditions: According to research, vitamin D may play a role in modifying autoimmune reactions. It has the potential to help modulate immunological responses that contribute to diseases such as multiple sclerosis, rheumatoid arthritis, and systemic lupus erythematosus.

5. Respiratory Health: The role of vitamin D in immune function is especially important in the context of respiratory health. Adequate vitamin D levels have been linked to a lower risk of respiratory illnesses including the flu and the common cold. Some research suggests that vitamin D may aid in the body's protection against respiratory infections.

6. Immunological System Balancing: Vitamin D aids in the maintenance of a balanced immunological response. It can improve the body's ability to respond

to infections while also limiting overly aggressive immune responses that can damage tissue.

7. Immunological Response Modulation: Vitamin D can impact the balance of different types of immunological responses. It aids in the regulation of immune cell development into subtypes that perform diverse tasks, such as stimulating inflammation or dampening immunological reactivity.

8. Seasonal Variation and Immunity: According to some research, lower vitamin D levels during the winter months, when sunlight exposure is reduced, may contribute to an increased susceptibility to infections. This seasonal change in immunological health is currently being studied.

9. Individual Variation: The effect of vitamin D on immunological function varies from person to person. Genetics, underlying health issues, and overall immune system health can all have an impact on how vitamin D influences immunological responses.

While the link between vitamin D and immune function appears to be promising, it is crucial to recognize that vitamin D is only one of several elements influencing immunological health. Maintaining a healthy diet, engaging in regular physical activity, getting adequate sleep, and controlling stress are all important for maintaining a strong immune system. If you have specific concerns about your immunological health or vitamin D levels, like with any health-related topic, it is best to visit a healthcare expert.

Vitamin D and Bone Health in Elderly People

Vitamin D is essential for sustaining bone health throughout life, and its value is amplified in older populations. As people age, their bone density decreases, increasing their risk of osteoporosis and fractures. Vitamin D is required for calcium absorption and bone mineralization, making it an important element in the prevention of bone-related disorders in the elderly. Here's how vitamin D affects bone health in the elderly:

1. Calcium Absorption: Vitamin D improves calcium absorption from the intestines into the circulation. This calcium is subsequently used for bone mineralization, which aids in bone density and strength maintenance.
2. Bone Mineralization: Adequate vitamin D levels are required for adequate calcium and phosphorus

deposition into the bone matrix. This mechanism keeps bones robust and resistant to fractures.

3. Osteoporosis Prevention: Osteoporosis is a disorder that causes weaker bones that are more susceptible to fractures. By supporting bone density and structure, maintaining appropriate vitamin D levels can help lower the incidence of osteoporosis.

4. Fracture Risk Reduction: Low bone density and bone strength increase the risk of fractures, particularly in the elderly. Adequate vitamin D levels, together with calcium consumption and other bone-healthy activities, can help reduce the incidence of fractures.

5. Muscular Function: Vitamin D is also important for muscular function. Strong muscles help to support bones and prevent falls, which can result in fractures. muscular weakness and poor balance are common problems in the elderly, and vitamin D may help to maintain muscular health.

6. Fall Prevention: Falls are a major issue for older people since they can result in fractures and other injuries. Adequate vitamin D levels, as well as physical activity and balance training, can help lower the risk of falling.

7. Supplemental Support: Older persons may have less sun exposure and a lower ability of their skin to manufacture vitamin D from sunshine. To establish optimal levels for bone health, vitamin D supplements may be advised. A consultation with a healthcare provider is required to determine the proper dosage.

8. When combined with calcium, vitamin D has a synergistic effect on bone health. Adequate consumption of these nutrients is critical for bone density maintenance and prevention of bone-related problems.

Maintaining bone health is critical for aging populations' overall well-being and mobility. A balanced diet, frequent physical activity, and other bone-healthy activities, coupled with optimal vitamin D intake, can help promote strong and resilient bones as people age.

Vitamin D and Chronic Pain

Vitamin D is well-known for its role in bone health, immune function, and several physiological functions. A new study is also looking into the potential link between vitamin D levels and chronic pain issues. While the specific mechanisms are still being investigated, there is some evidence to suggest that maintaining appropriate vitamin D levels may aid in the management of chronic pain. What you should know about the vitamin D-chronic pain relationship:

1. Inflammatory Modulation: Anti-inflammatory effects of vitamin D may influence chronic pain syndromes defined by inflammation. Inflammation is linked to a variety of pain disorders, and vitamin D's impacts on the immune system and inflammation pathways may help with pain alleviation.

2. Nerve Function and Pain Perception: Vitamin D has been linked to nerve function and transmission. Adequate vitamin D levels may aid in the maintenance of good nerve health and the reduction of nerve-related pain symptoms.

3. Musculoskeletal Health: Vitamin D's role in bone and muscle health can have an impact on chronic pain problems involving musculoskeletal issues, such as osteoarthritis, fibromyalgia, and back pain.

4. Neuropathic Pain: Neuropathic pain is characterized by nerve-related pain sensations and is frequently difficult to treat. According to some studies, vitamin

D insufficiency may be associated with an increased risk of neuropathic pain problems.

5. Immune System Interactions: Immune system dysfunction can have an impact on chronic pain problems. The significance of vitamin D in immune modulation and its possible impact on immune-related pain pathways are being studied.

6. Pain Perception and Mood: Chronic pain can have a substantial impact on mental health. According to new research, maintaining optimal vitamin D levels may be related to enhanced mood, which may alter pain perception indirectly.

While research into the potential link between vitamin D and chronic pain reduction is ongoing, vitamin D supplements should not be used in place of other recognized pain management strategies or medical therapies. Chronic pain is a complicated condition, and it's important to collaborate with healthcare specialists to build a thorough and tailored pain treatment strategy.

The Benefits of Vitamin D

Vitamin D, also known as the "sunshine vitamin," is an essential mineral with numerous health and wellness advantages. It is essential in many physiological processes and is important for more than simply bone health. Here are some of the most important vitamin D benefits:

1. Health of the Bones: Calcium absorption and bone mineralization require vitamin D. It aids in the maintenance of strong and healthy bones, lowering the risk of disorders like osteoporosis and fractures.

2. Support for the Immune System: Vitamin D modifies the immune system, allowing it to respond more effectively to infections and disorders. Adequate intake of vitamin D helps to improve immune function.

3. Inflammation Control: Vitamin D has anti-inflammatory effects that can help modulate the inflammatory response in the body. It may help in the management of chronic inflammatory disorders.

4. Muscle Function: Maintaining healthy muscles requires adequate vitamin D levels. Muscle weakness and reduced function can result from a lack of vitamin D.

5. Cardiovascular Health: According to some studies, adequate vitamin D levels may benefit cardiovascular health by encouraging appropriate blood pressure levels and lowering the risk of heart disease.

6. Mood and Mental Health: Vitamin D is associated with mood management and mental health. Low vitamin D levels have been linked to a higher risk of mood disorders such as depression and anxiety.

7. Cancer Prevention: While further research is needed, several studies suggest that maintaining adequate vitamin D levels may relate to a lower risk of some malignancies such as breast, prostate, colorectal, and pancreatic cancer.

8. Diabetes Treatment: Vitamin D may help with insulin sensitivity and glucose metabolism. According to some research, optimal vitamin D levels may assist diabetics maintain their blood sugar levels.

9. Autoimmune Disorders: Emerging research reveals a link between vitamin D insufficiency and autoimmune illnesses such as multiple sclerosis, rheumatoid arthritis, and type 1 diabetes.

10. Respiratory Health: Adequate vitamin D levels have been linked to a lower incidence of respiratory infections and better lung function. Vitamin D may help improve respiratory health.

11. Pregnancy and Fetal Development: Vitamin D is essential for the health of both the mother and the fetus during pregnancy. It promotes appropriate fetal

bone growth and lowers the incidence of problems such as preeclampsia.

12.   Neurological Health: Some research suggests that vitamin D may play a role in neurological health and cognitive function, perhaps lowering the risk of illnesses such as Alzheimer's disease.

13.   Lifespan and Aging: Maintaining appropriate vitamin D levels is linked to healthy aging and lifespan. It promotes a variety of body functions that contribute to overall health as you age.

It's crucial to understand that, while vitamin D has various benefits, too much of it can be hazardous. Before making large changes to your vitamin D intake, especially through supplementation, you should see a healthcare expert. To gain its many benefits, it is critical to strike a balance between proper vitamin D levels, sun safety, and general health habits.

CHAPTER THREE: VITAMIN C THE IMMUNITY SUPPLEMENT

Introduction of Vitamin C

Vitamin C, commonly known as ascorbic acid, is a water-soluble vitamin that is essential for the body's growth, development, and function. It is essential for the manufacturing of collagen, an important protein that aids in wound healing, blood vessel strengthening, and the maintenance of healthy skin, bones, and teeth.

Vitamin C is also a potent antioxidant, which means it helps protect bodily cells from free radical damage. Free radicals are unstable chemicals that can cause chronic diseases like cancer, heart disease, and premature aging. Vitamin C can help prevent or reduce the progression of many diseases by neutralizing free radicals.

Furthermore, vitamin C improves iron absorption from plant-based meals. Iron is required for the formation of red blood cells, which are responsible for transporting oxygen throughout the body. It also helps the immune system by boosting the creation of white blood cells, which fight infections.

Because the human body cannot generate or store vitamin C, it must be received from diet or supplementation. Citrus fruits (such as oranges and grapefruits), strawberries, kiwi, bell peppers, broccoli, tomatoes, and leafy green vegetables are all high in vitamin C. The recommended daily consumption of vitamin C varies according to age, gender, and stage of life. The recommended daily dose for adults is typically 75-90 mg per day. However, higher doses may be advised in specific circumstances, such as during pregnancy or for smokers, as smoking can decrease vitamin C levels in the body.

Fatigue, weakness, bleeding gums, joint and muscular problems, and poor wound healing are all symptoms of vitamin C insufficiency.

Finally, vitamin C is a necessary ingredient that aids in a variety of bodily activities such as collagen formation, antioxidant protection, iron absorption, and immune system support. To maintain maximum health and prevent deficiencies, it is critical to get enough vitamin C through a balanced diet or supplements.

Sources of Vitamin C

Vitamin C is abundant in many fruits and vegetables, making it simple to integrate into your diet. Here are some excellent vitamin C dietary sources:

1. Citrus Fruits: Citrus fruits are one of the most well-known sources of vitamin C. Oranges, tangerines, limes, lemons, and grapefruits are all examples of citrus fruits.
2. Berries: Berries have very high antioxidants and vitamin C. Strawberries, blackberries, blueberries, and raspberries are types of berries.
3. Kiwi: Kiwi is high in vitamin C. It also contains a lot of fiber and other nutrients.
4. Bell peppers: Bell peppers, particularly the red and yellow types, are high in vitamin C. They go well in salads, stir-fries, and other foods.
5. Broccoli: Broccoli is a vegetable and is also another source of vitamin C. It also contains other vitamins and minerals as well.
6. Brussels Sprouts: Brussels sprouts are another cruciferous vegetable that is high in vitamin C and has numerous health advantages.

7. Pineapple: A tropical fruit high in vitamin C, pineapple also includes an enzyme called bromelain, which may offer extra health advantages.

8. Mango: Not only is mango sweet, but it is also high in vitamin C and other nutrients.

9. Papaya: Papaya is a tropical fruit that is high in vitamin C and also high in enzymes and antioxidants.

10. Cantaloupe: A type of melon, cantaloupe is a delicious source of vitamin C, especially during the summer months.

11. Tomatoes: Tomatoes, whether fresh or in tomato products (such as tomato sauce or canned tomatoes), are high in vitamin C.

12. Leafy Greens: Leafy greens such as spinach, kale, and Swiss chard contain vitamin C as well, albeit in slightly lower amounts than some fruits.

13. Guava: Guava is a tropical fruit that is rich in vitamin C and contains fiber.

14. Acerola Cherry: Acerola cherry, commonly known as Barbados cherry, is a high-quality natural source of vitamin C.

15. Fortified Foods: Some foods, such as cereals and beverages, are fortified with vitamin C to provide an extra boost.

Consuming a range of vitamin C-rich foods will help you satisfy your daily vitamin requirements. Keep in mind that cooking methods can have an impact on the vitamin C content of foods, with some loss occurring during the cooking process. Consider eating some of these foods fresh or with minimal preparation to retain the most vitamin C. Consult a healthcare practitioner or qualified dietitian for specialized advice on incorporating vitamin C-rich foods into your diet if you have dietary limitations, allergies, or other health problems.

Vitamin C Functions

Vitamin C performs various important activities in the body. It is a necessary nutrient that aids in a variety of physiological functions, contributing to general health and well-being. Some important functions of vitamin C are:

1. Antioxidant Defense

   Antioxidants are chemicals that protect cells from oxidative stress and damage caused by dangerous molecules known as free radicals. Vitamin C, commonly known as ascorbic acid, is a powerful antioxidant that protects the body from oxidative damage throughout the body. As an antioxidant, vitamin C works as follows:

a. Scavenging of Free Radicals: Free radicals are extremely reactive chemicals that can harm cells, DNA, and other biological components. Vitamin C serves as a free radical scavenger, contributing an electron to stabilize them. This procedure protects free radicals from damaging cells.

b. Cellular Protection: The antioxidant capabilities of vitamin C help protect cells from oxidative stress, which can lead to cellular malfunction, inflammation, and a variety of chronic diseases.

c. Lipid Protection: Oxidative stress can cause lipids (fats) in cell membranes to be damaged, resulting in cellular malfunction. Vitamin C aids in the prevention of lipid peroxidation, a process that damages cell membranes and contributes to a variety of health problems.

d. DNA Preservation: Oxidative damage to DNA can cause mutations, which can lead to the development of cancer and other disorders. The antioxidant activity of vitamin C aids in the preservation of DNA integrity.

e. Immune System Support: As part of their defense processes, immune cells produce reactive oxygen species (ROS). Vitamin C regulates the balance of ROS and antioxidants within immune cells, preventing excessive oxidative stress.

f. Antioxidant Regeneration: Vitamin C has the unusual capacity to renew other antioxidants, such as vitamin E. When vitamin E neutralizes a free radical, it undergoes oxidation. Vitamin C can rebuild oxidized vitamin E, allowing it to continue to function as an antioxidant.

g. Collaboration with Other Antioxidants: Vitamin C collaborates with other antioxidants like vitamin E, glutathione, and selenium. These antioxidants work together to provide full protection against oxidative damage.

h. Skin Health: The antioxidant properties of vitamin C are especially useful to skin health. It shields skin cells from UV rays, pollution, and other environmental factors that can hasten skin aging.

i. Disease Prevention: Chronic diseases such as heart disease, cancer, diabetes, and neurological disorders have been related to oxidative stress. The antioxidant effect of vitamin C may help to reduce the risk of several disorders.

j. Improved Plant-Based Iron Absorption: Vitamin C improves the absorption of non-heme iron (the iron contained in plant-based diets). Because iron can generate free radicals in excess, this helps the body's total antioxidant defense.

Consuming a range of vitamin C-rich meals and maintaining appropriate vitamin C levels can help to provide effective antioxidant protection. Vitamin C is abundant in fruits and vegetables, particularly those that are colored. It's crucial to note, however, that taking too many vitamin C supplements may not deliver any additional benefits and may perhaps have the opposite impact. As with any dietary decision, it's advisable to seek specific advice from a healthcare practitioner for maintaining a balanced antioxidant-rich diet.

2. Collagen Production

Collagen is the most prevalent protein in the human body and is an important structural component of many tissues such as skin, bones, tendons, ligaments, and blood vessels. Vitamin C is essential for collagen synthesis, which is the process of forming and assembling collagen molecules into fibers. Here's how vitamin C helps in collagen synthesis:

a. Proline and Lysine Hydroxylation: Collagen is made up of amino acids, the most essential of which are proline and lysine. Vitamin C is required for the hydroxylation (addition of hydroxyl groups) of proline and lysine residues in the polypeptide chains of collagen. This hydroxylation is essential for the stability of collagen's triple helix structure.

b. Triple Helix Formation: Collagen molecules are made up of three polypeptide chains that are linked together in a triple helix configuration. Vitamin C-mediated hydroxylation of proline and lysine residues aids in the stability of this structure, allowing collagen molecules to align and bond securely together.

c. Collagen Fiber Cross-Linking: Collagen fibers are further stabilized through cross-linking, a process that improves tissue strength and durability. The role of vitamin C in collagen production aids in the development of these cross-links.

d. Tissue Formation and Repair: Collagen is a protein that is found in many tissues, including skin, cartilage, bones, and blood vessels. The structural integrity of these tissues is ensured by proper collagen synthesis, which also aids in tissue creation and repair.

e. Skin Health: Collagen is an important component of the extracellular matrix of the skin, providing strength and suppleness. Adequate collagen production, aided by vitamin C, contributes to youthful-looking skin.

f. Wound Healing: The role of vitamin C in collagen formation is especially crucial for wound healing. Collagen provides scaffolding for tissue repair, and enough collagen synthesis speeds up the healing process.

g. Blood Vessel Integrity: Collagen is found in blood vessel walls, where it contributes to their strength and flexibility. The effect of vitamin C on collagen formation indirectly benefits cardiovascular health by preserving blood vessel integrity.

h. Bone Health: Collagen is also found in the bone matrix, where it serves as a scaffolding for mineralization. While vitamin C plays a more direct function in collagen synthesis, it also indirectly contributes to bone health by supporting collagen's structural role in bone development.

i. Connective Tissue Function: Collagen is essential for the formation and function of many connective tissues in the body, including tendons and ligaments. The strength and flexibility of these tissues are ensured by proper collagen synthesis, which is aided by vitamin C.

Inadequate vitamin C levels can inhibit collagen formation and, in severe situations, result in scurvy. Scurvy symptoms include bleeding gums, joint pain, weariness, and delayed wound healing. Consuming vitamin C-rich meals like fruits and vegetables is critical for maintaining normal collagen synthesis and general health. If you have special health issues or dietary restrictions, a healthcare practitioner or qualified dietitian can provide tailored advice on reaching your vitamin C requirements.

3. Wound Repair

Wound healing is a complex process that involves numerous cellular and biochemical systems that collaborate to mend injured tissues. Vitamin C is essential in wound healing because it supports these processes and promotes the rapid regeneration of wounded tissue. The following is how vitamin C aids in wound healing:

a. Tissue Formation: New tissue must be formed during wound healing to replace injured or lost tissue. The role of vitamin C in collagen production aids in the development of new connective tissue, promoting wound closure.

b. Angiogenesis: Angiogenesis is the process through which new blood vessels are formed. Adequate vitamin C levels are required for this process because new blood vessels give oxygen and nutrients to the wound site, assisting in tissue repair.

c. Immune Function: Vitamin C helps the immune system, which is important during wound healing to avoid infection. It helps to regulate inflammation at the wound site and boosts the body's defense mechanisms.

d. Cell Proliferation: Wound healing requires the proliferation and migration of numerous cells, including fibroblasts, which make collagen, and keratinocytes, which build the skin's outer layer. Vitamin C promotes tissue repair by increasing cell proliferation.

e. Epithelialization: Epithelialization is the process by which the wound is covered by the skin's outermost layer (epidermis). Vitamin C promotes keratinocyte migration, which aids in the repair of the epidermal barrier.

f. Scar Formation: Scar formation is aided by collagen created during wound healing. Proper collagen synthesis, aided by vitamin C, contributes to scar tissue that is robust and resilient.

g. Wound Contraction: Vitamin C may help with wound contraction, which is the process by which the edges of a wound come together. This contraction shrinks the wound and speeds up healing.

h. Cellular Communication: Vitamin C participates in several cellular signaling pathways that control wound healing, ensuring coordinated and effective repair.

It is vital to highlight that a lack of vitamin C might affect wound healing, resulting in delayed or ineffective recovery. Adequate vitamin C intake from a balanced diet that includes vitamin C-rich foods like fruits and vegetables is critical for effective wound healing. Healthcare practitioners may recommend supplemental vitamin C dosage to support appropriate tissue regeneration in cases of major wounds, operations, or medical problems that impact wound healing. Consult a healthcare provider for specific advice if you have concerns regarding wound healing or are considering supplementing.

4. Immune System Support

Vitamin C is well-known for its involvement in immune system support, which is vital in fighting the body against infections and disorders. The immune-boosting actions of vitamin C are diverse, contributing to numerous facets of immune function. Here are some ways vitamin C can help your immune system:

a. Improved White Blood Cell Function: Vitamin C aids in the generation and function of white blood cells such as neutrophils, lymphocytes, and phagocytes. These cells play an important role in the immune system because they help identify and remove pathogens such as bacteria and viruses.

b. Antioxidant Protection: Vitamin C is a powerful antioxidant that protects immune cells from oxidative damage caused by free radicals. This antioxidant defense ensures that immune cells operate properly.

c. Immune Cell Maturation: Vitamin C aids in the maturation of specific immune cells. It promotes immune cell differentiation and development to enable optimal immune response performance.

d. Immune Tissue Collagen Synthesis: Immune cells and tissues, such as lymph nodes and the thymus, rely on collagen for structural integrity. The role of vitamin C in collagen formation contributes to the strength and functionality of these immune-related structures.

e. Cytokine Synthesis: Vitamin C can influence cytokine synthesis, which is a signaling molecule that regulates immunological responses. This regulation aids in the maintenance of a balanced immune response.

f. Barrier Function: Vitamin C helps to maintain the skin and mucosal barrier, which functions as a physical barrier against pathogens. Healthy skin and mucosal membranes are the first line of protection against infections.

g. Viral Infections: Vitamin C has been examined for its antiviral properties. It may help to lessen the severity and duration of viral diseases like the common cold and influenza.

h. Immune System Training: The influence of vitamin C on immune cell function can help support a properly trained immunological response. This means that the immune system can recognize and respond to viruses more effectively.

i. Stress Response: Vitamin C levels may be decreased during times of physical or emotional stress. Adequate vitamin C intake is essential for immune system maintenance during times of elevated demand.

Maintaining adequate vitamin C levels through a balanced diet rich in vitamin C-rich foods like fruits and vegetables is critical for good immune function. While vitamin C can help with immunological function, it is not a cure-all for avoiding or treating illnesses. Consult a healthcare expert for individualized suggestions if you have specific health concerns or are contemplating vitamin C supplements for immune support.

5. Iron Absorption

Vitamin C is essential for the absorption of non-heme iron, which is found in plant-based diets and iron-fortified products. This interaction is especially relevant for vegetarians and vegans because non-heme iron is often less readily absorbed than heme iron from animal sources. This is how vitamin C aids iron absorption:

a. Reducing Iron to Its Ferrous Form: Iron is frequently contained in plant-based meals in its ferric (Fe^{3+}) form, which is less readily absorbed by the body. Vitamin C aids in the conversion of ferric iron to ferrous (Fe^{2+}) iron, which is more soluble and easier for the body to absorb.

b. Iron Chelation: In the digestive tract, vitamin C forms a complex with iron, increasing its solubility and preventing it from interacting with substances that restrict absorption, such as phytates and tannins.

c. Transport via the Intestinal Wall: Iron's enhanced solubility because of its interaction with vitamin C allows it to pass past the intestinal wall and into the bloodstream, where it can be transported to numerous tissues.

d. Improved Absorption Efficiency: Because of vitamin C's effect on iron absorption, non-heme iron is absorbed more efficiently. This can help those who rely on plant-based iron sources to achieve their iron requirements.

e. Increased Iron Availability: Vitamin C helps guarantee that iron is more readily available for the body's physiological activities, such as hemoglobin and myoglobin formation, by enhancing non-heme iron absorption.

f. Iron Deficiency Anemia: Iron deficiency anemia is a frequent illness defined by low iron levels in the body, resulting in decreased red blood cell synthesis. Adequate vitamin C consumption can help prevent or treat iron deficiency anemia.

g. Plant-Based Diets That Are Balanced: Vegetarian and vegan diets can be deficient in readily absorbable iron. Iron absorption and iron balance can be improved by eating vitamin C-rich foods alongside iron-rich plant foods.

To maximize the advantages of vitamin C on iron absorption, combine iron-rich plant foods (such as beans, lentils, spinach, and fortified cereals) with vitamin C-rich foods (such as citrus fruits, bell peppers, and broccoli) while eating.

It is vital to note that excessive vitamin C consumption will not result in excessive iron absorption over the body's requirements. Instead, vitamin C aids iron absorption in people who would otherwise struggle to absorb adequate iron from plant-based sources. If you have special iron-related issues, dietary limitations, or medical problems, you should get tailored advice from a healthcare expert or qualified dietitian on maximizing your iron intake and absorption.

6. Neurotransmitter Production

Vitamin C aids in the manufacture and function of neurotransmitters, which are chemical messengers that send impulses between nerve cells (neurons) in the brain and throughout the nervous system. These neurotransmitters are critical for mood, cognition, and a variety of physiological activities. Here's how vitamin C affects neurotransmitter production:

a. Dopamine Synthesis: Vitamin C is essential for the conversion of tyrosine, an amino acid, into dopamine, a neurotransmitter involved in motivation, reward, pleasure, and mood regulation. Dopamine is also involved in the regulation of locomotion.

b. Synthesis of Norepinephrine: Vitamin C is also required for the conversion of dopamine to norepinephrine (noradrenaline). Norepinephrine has a role in the "fight or flight" reaction, as well as alertness and stress response.

c. Epinephrine Synthesis: Norepinephrine is converted into epinephrine (adrenaline), and vitamin C aids in this process. Epinephrine is a neurotransmitter and hormone that plays an important part in the body's response to stress and emergency.

d. Serotonin Synthesis: While vitamin C is not directly involved in serotonin synthesis, it indirectly supports it by sustaining the enzymatic conversion of tryptophan (an amino acid) into serotonin. Serotonin, also known as the "feel-good" neurotransmitter, is linked to mood control, sleep, and appetite.

e. Balance of Neurotransmitters: Adequate vitamin C levels contribute to optimal mood control, cognitive function, and overall mental well-being by maintaining the balance of neurotransmitters.

f. Neurotransmitter Release: The antioxidant characteristics of vitamin C can protect neurons and neurotransmitter receptors from oxidative damage, resulting in effective neurotransmitter release and communication.

g. Cognitive Function: Neurotransmitters play an important role in cognitive activities such as memory, learning, attention, and problem-solving. The effect of vitamin C in neurotransmitter synthesis indirectly benefits cognitive function.

h. Stress Response: Vitamin C influences the creation and balance of neurotransmitters, which can affect the body's response to stress and emotional challenges.

i. Mood management: Vitamin C's role in neurotransmitter synthesis and balance can have an effect on mood management. Low vitamin C levels have been linked to mood disorders such as depression.

j. Neuromuscular Function: Neurotransmitters are necessary for nerve cell and muscle communication. Vitamin C helps to maintain appropriate neuromuscular activity in an indirect way.

A balanced diet with optimal vitamin C levels contributes to the generation and balance of neurotransmitters, which supports mood, cognition, and overall nervous system function. Vitamin C, on the other hand, is just one of several elements that regulate neurotransmitter production, and its effects on mental health are complex. If you have specific mental health difficulties or are considering supplementation, it is best to seek specialized advice from a healthcare expert.

7. Bone Health

While vitamin C's impact on bone health is not as significant as it is in collagen production and antioxidant protection, it nevertheless serves a supportive role in the maintenance of strong and healthy bones. Here's how vitamin C helps with bone health:

a. Formation of Collagen: Collagen is a major component of the bone matrix, providing the structural underpinning for bones. Vitamin C is required for collagen synthesis, which adds to bone strength, flexibility, and general integrity.

b. Bone Mineralization: Vitamin C indirectly aids bone mineralization by encouraging the development of collagen fibers, which serve as a scaffold for minerals such as calcium and phosphorus.

c. Connective Tissue Support: Connective tissues such as tendons, ligaments, and cartilage, in addition to bones, are crucial for general bone health. The significance of vitamin C in collagen formation benefits the health and function of these connective tissues.

d. Wound Healing and Bone Repair: The role of vitamin C in wound healing is also important for bone health. Collagen production is required for tissue repair and regeneration in properly healed bone fractures and traumas.

e. Antioxidant Protection: Oxidative stress can harm bone health by interfering with bone remodeling and leading to bone loss. The antioxidant properties of vitamin C aid in the prevention of oxidative damage and the maintenance of bone health.

f. Osteoclast and Osteoblast Function: Vitamin C has the potential to alter the activity of osteoclasts (cells that tear down bone tissue) and osteoblasts (cells that produce new bone tissue) by influencing the synthesis of signaling molecules involved in bone remodeling.

g. Bone Density and Fracture Risk: Adequate vitamin C levels may help to maintain bone density and reduce fracture risk, particularly when combined with other bone-supportive nutrients like calcium and vitamin D.

h. Strength of the Collagen Network: The collagen network in bone tissue provides resilience and shock absorption. The significance of vitamin C in collagen formation adds to the overall strength and durability of this network.

i. Age-Related Bone Health: Due to the natural reduction in bone density, bone health becomes a key concern as people age. Maintaining enough vitamin C levels can benefit bone health as we age.

While vitamin C is beneficial to bone health, additional minerals such as calcium, vitamin D, magnesium, and vitamin K are also required for optimal bone health. A well-balanced diet rich in nutrient-dense foods is essential for maintaining overall bone health. Consultation with a healthcare expert or qualified dietitian can provide individualized advice on keeping strong and healthy bones if you have specific concerns about bone health, dietary issues, or underlying medical disorders.

8. Cardiovascular Health

Vitamin C contributes to cardiovascular health by supporting numerous systems that promote the healthy functioning of the circulatory system. While vitamin C is not a cure for heart disease, its effects can supplement a healthy lifestyle to enhance heart health. Here's how vitamin C affects cardiovascular health:

a. Antioxidant Protection: Vitamin C is a powerful antioxidant that helps protect cells, blood vessels, and cardiac tissues from free radical oxidative damage. Reducing oxidative stress may help to prevent cardiovascular disease.

b. Blood Vessel Health: Vitamin C promotes blood vessel health by promoting its integrity and elasticity. This can aid in the prevention of problems such as atherosclerosis (artery hardening) and the maintenance of appropriate blood pressure.

c. Endothelial Function: The endothelium, or inner lining of blood vessels, regulates blood vessel tone and blood flow. Adequate vitamin C levels promote endothelial function, which is essential for cardiovascular health.

d. Nitric Oxide synthesis: Vitamin C aids in the synthesis of nitric oxide, a chemical that aids in the relaxation of blood vessels and the improvement of blood flow. Healthy nitric oxide levels help to keep blood pressure in check.

e. Collagen Synthesis in Blood Vessels: Collagen is found in blood vessel walls and adds to their strength and structure. The significance of vitamin C in collagen formation promotes the health and integrity of blood vessels.

f. Reduction of Inflammation: Chronic inflammation is a risk factor for cardiovascular disease. The antioxidant properties of vitamin C may aid in reducing inflammation and lowering the risk of developing heart disease.

g. Cholesterol Levels: Some research suggests that vitamin C consumption relates to reduced levels of LDL cholesterol (often known as "bad" cholesterol) and total cholesterol, which can help with cardiovascular health.

h. Blood Clotting: By suppressing platelet aggregation, vitamin C may help prevent excessive blood clotting. This may lower the incidence of clot-related problems such as heart attacks and strokes.

i. Blood Sugar Regulation: Vitamin C consumption has been linked to enhanced glucose metabolism, which can aid in blood

> sugar management and lower the risk of diabetes-related cardiovascular problems.
>
> j. Support for Collateral Circulation: Collateral circulation refers to the formation of new blood vessels that can compensate for reduced blood flow. The importance of vitamin C in blood vessel health promotes the establishment of these alternate routes.

While vitamin C is a key contributor to cardiovascular health, it is critical to address heart health holistically. A heart-healthy lifestyle includes eating a balanced diet, maintaining a healthy weight, engaging in regular physical activity, managing stress, avoiding smoking, and monitoring blood pressure and cholesterol levels. If you have pre-existing cardiovascular issues or concerns, it is best to talk with a healthcare practitioner to build a specific strategy for promoting cardiovascular health.

9. Antiviral and antimicrobial properties

Vitamin C has been investigated for its antiviral and antibacterial properties. While vitamin C is not a substitute for medical treatment, its immune-supporting characteristics and influence on diverse immunological activities contribute to its role in improving infection defense. Here's how vitamin C can help fight viruses and bacteria:

a. Immune System Support: Vitamin C is essential for the immune system, which serves as the body's protection against illnesses. A healthy immune system aids in the detection and elimination of viruses, germs, and other infections.

b. Improved Immune Cell activity: Vitamin C aids in the generation and activity of white blood cells such as neutrophils, lymphocytes, and phagocytes, all of which play important roles in the immune response to infections.

c. Viral Replication is Reduced: Some research suggests that vitamin C may interfere with the replication of certain viruses. While the processes are unknown, vitamin C's antioxidant capabilities and influence on immunological responses may play a role.

d. Reduced Illness Duration: Vitamin C supplementation has been linked to a reduction in the duration and intensity of typical cold symptoms. While it is not a cure, it may assist in relieving symptoms and promoting the body's ability to heal.

e. Cytokine Modulation: Vitamin C can alter the synthesis and function of cytokines, which are signaling molecules that govern immune responses. A well-coordinated immune response is supported by proper cytokine balance.

f. Direct Antiviral Benefits: Although vitamin C may have direct antiviral benefits against certain viruses, their effects are often weaker when compared to antiviral drugs.

g. Synergistic Effects: The immune-boosting properties of vitamin C can supplement other antiviral and antimicrobial measures such as immunization, appropriate hygiene, and medical therapies.

h. Wound Healing and Infection Prevention: The role of vitamin C in wound healing is related to infection prevention. Proper wound healing avoids pathogen entrance and promotes immune responses at the site of injury.

While vitamin C can help with immune function, it is not a foolproof technique for avoiding or curing illnesses. Before using vitamin C supplements or making large dietary changes, consult with a healthcare provider, especially if you have underlying health concerns or are using drugs.

10.   Skin Health

Vitamin C, often known as ascorbic acid, is essential for keeping skin healthy. Its antioxidant capabilities, role in collagen formation, and other actions all help the overall health of the skin. Vitamin C can help your skin in the following ways:

a. Collagen creation: Vitamin C is required for the creation of collagen, a protein that gives the skin and other tissues structural support. Collagen promotes skin elasticity, firmness, and a young appearance.

b. Wound Healing: Collagen is essential for wound healing because it serves as a scaffolding for tissue repair. Adequate vitamin C levels are required for wound healing, which includes the development of new skin tissue.

c. Antioxidant Protection: The antioxidant capabilities of vitamin C help protect skin cells from oxidative stress produced by UV radiation, pollution, and other environmental conditions.

This protection can help to halt the aging process and lower the chance of skin injury.

d. Skin Barrier Function: Vitamin C helps to maintain the skin's barrier function, which keeps moisture in and dangerous bacteria and irritants out. Maintaining moisturized and bright skin requires a strong skin barrier.

e. Collagen Stabilization: Vitamin C helps to stabilize collagen molecules, allowing them to assemble and function properly within the skin. This helps to maintain the skin's general integrity and strength.

f. Skin Brightening and Even Tone: Vitamin C prevents the synthesis of melanin, the pigment that causes skin darkening. This feature can aid in the reduction of dark spots and the promotion of a more even skin tone.

g. Improved Sun Protection: The antioxidant properties of vitamin C can help the skin's natural defense against UV-induced damage. While not a replacement for sunscreen, using vitamin C-rich skincare products can provide additional protection.

h. Hydration Support: Vitamin C promotes the development of skin barrier lipids, which aids in moisture retention. This helps to give the skin a moisturized and plump appearance.

i. Elastin Creation: Vitamin C is also involved in the creation of elastin, another protein that helps to maintain skin elasticity. Healthy elastin strands help the skin snap back into place after being stretched.

j. Anti-Inflammatory Effects: The anti-inflammatory qualities of vitamin C can help reduce skin inflammation and redness, resulting in a calmer complexion.

k. Scarring and Hyperpigmentation: Because vitamin C aids in collagen formation, it can aid in scar healing and lessen the appearance of hyperpigmentation, such as acne scars.

l. Hyaluronic Acid creation: Vitamin C promotes the creation of hyaluronic acid, a chemical that aids in the maintenance of skin hydration and plumpness.

Incorporating vitamin C-rich foods into your diet and utilizing vitamin C-containing skincare products can help enhance skin health. A thorough skincare routine that includes sunscreen, regular washing, and moisturization is also essential for preserving healthy skin. If you have specific skin concerns or are thinking about utilizing vitamin C supplements or skincare products, talking with a dermatologist or skincare specialist can provide customized advice.

11.   Mood Control

Vitamin C, commonly known as ascorbic acid, is involved in several metabolic activities that may help with mood management and mental health. While vitamin C is not a direct treatment for mood disorders, its impact on neurotransmitters, oxidative stress, and overall brain function may help with emotional and mental wellness. Here are some possible effects of vitamin C on mood regulation:

a. Synthesis of Neurotransmitters: Vitamin C is necessary to produce neurotransmitters such as dopamine, norepinephrine, and serotonin. These neurotransmitters are essential for mood modulation, emotion regulation, and cognitive function.

b. Dopamine and Reward Pathways: Adequate vitamin C levels promote dopamine synthesis, a neurotransmitter involved with pleasure, motivation, and reward. Dopamine levels that are balanced contribute to a pleasant mood.

c. Norepinephrine and Alertness: Vitamin C also aids in the conversion of dopamine into norepinephrine, a neurotransmitter involved in alertness, focus, and the body's stress response.

d. Serotonin and Happiness: While vitamin C does not directly contribute to serotonin synthesis, it does aid in the conversion of tryptophan (an amino acid) to serotonin. Serotonin levels that are adequate are related to feelings of well-being and a happy mood.

e. Antioxidant Protection: The antioxidant properties of vitamin C help protect brain cells from oxidative damage. Reduced oxidative stress can aid in the maintenance of normal brain function and emotional well-being.

f. Reducing Neuroinflammation: Chronic inflammation in the brain has been linked to mood problems. The antioxidant properties of vitamin C can help reduce neuroinflammation, potentially supporting a healthy emotional state.

g. Stress Response: The action of vitamin C on neurotransmitters and its role in adrenal function may help with stress management and lower the detrimental impact of chronic stress on mood.

h. Cognitive Function: Mood and cognitive function are inextricably linked. Vitamin C indirectly adds to cognitive well-being by supporting neurotransmitter generation and overall brain health.

i. Hormone modulation: Vitamin C has been linked to hormone modulation, especially hormones associated with mood and stress response.

j. Collagen and Self-Image: While vitamin C does not directly affect mood, its role in collagen production can contribute to positive self-image and overall emotional well-being.

While vitamin C is one of many factors that influence mood and mental health, eating a balanced diet and keeping optimal amounts of this nutrient can help with general well-being. However, vitamin C alone is not a replacement for skilled mental health care. If you are having mood problems or other mental health issues, it is critical that you seek the advice of a mental health expert, such as a therapist or psychiatrist. They can give accurate diagnosis, therapy, and support that is targeted to your specific needs.

12.   Metabolism

Vitamin C, commonly known as ascorbic acid, is involved in a variety of metabolic activities in the body. While vitamin C is not a miraculous weight reduction or metabolism booster, its impacts on energy production, antioxidant defense, and overall health all contribute to its involvement in metabolism. Here's how vitamin C affects metabolism:

a. Energy Production: Vitamin C is essential for the manufacture of carnitine, a molecule that aids in the transport of fatty acids into the mitochondria, the energy-producing centers of the cell. This procedure is required for the conversion of fat to energy.

b. Antioxidant Defense: The antioxidant capabilities of vitamin C aid in the protection of cells from oxidative stress induced by metabolic processes and environmental stimuli. Reducing oxidative stress benefits cellular health and energy generation in general.

c. Collagen production: Collagen production is crucial not just for the skin and connective tissues, but also for metabolic activities. Collagen helps to maintain the structural integrity of blood arteries, which are necessary for the delivery of nutrients and oxygen to cells.

d. Hormone Regulation: Vitamin C may play a function in hormone regulation, particularly metabolism and energy balance hormones.

e. Iron Absorption: As previously stated, vitamin C aids in the absorption of non-heme iron from plant-based diets. Iron levels must be enough for oxygen delivery and energy synthesis.

f. Carnitine Biosynthesis: Carnitine aids in the transport of fatty acids into mitochondria, where they are converted into energy. Vitamin C aids in the manufacture of carnitine, which influences fat metabolism indirectly.

g. Immune Support: A healthy immune system is essential for general health and metabolism. The immune-boosting effects of vitamin C help to keep metabolic processes running smoothly.

h. Collateral Circulation: In the context of metabolism, vitamin C's role in stimulating the development of collateral circulation (alternative blood vessel paths) can aid in the transport of nutrients and oxygen to tissues.

i. Cellular Communication: Effective cellular communication is essential for metabolic processes. The effect of vitamin C on neurotransmitter production and function can influence metabolic cellular signaling.

j. Detoxification: The antioxidant properties of vitamin C can help the body's detoxification activities by neutralizing toxic compounds created during metabolism.

While vitamin C aids metabolism, it is critical to approach weight control and overall health through a holistic strategy that includes a balanced diet, frequent physical activity, good hydration, and adequate sleep. There is no "magic bullet" for losing weight or boosting metabolism. If you're thinking about using vitamin C supplements for metabolic assistance, make sure they're compatible with your overall health goals and medical needs.

13.   Dental Health

Vitamin C, commonly known as ascorbic acid, is not only important for overall health but also for optimum oral health. Its impacts on collagen formation, wound healing, immunological support, and antioxidant protection all help to improve dental health. Here's how vitamin C can help your teeth:

a. Collagen production: Vitamin C is required for collagen production, a protein that creates the structural underpinning of connective tissues such as gums. Gum health is critical for tooth stability and general oral health.

b. Gum Health: Adequate vitamin C levels promote gum tissue health and integrity. A vitamin C deficiency can cause gum bleeding, inflammation (gingivitis), and more serious gum disease (periodontitis).

c. Wound Healing: Vitamin C is required for wound healing, particularly gum tissue healing after dental operations or injuries. Proper wound healing keeps germs and pathogens out.

d. Immune Support: Vitamin C's immune-boosting qualities aid the body's defenses against infections, particularly oral infections. It aids the body's defense against microorganisms that cause tooth decay and gum disease.

e. Antioxidant Protection: The antioxidant properties of vitamin C serve to protect oral tissues from oxidative stress caused by damaging free radicals. Gum inflammation and oral tissue damage can be exacerbated by oxidative stress.

f. Collagen Stabilization: Vitamin C aids in the stabilization of collagen molecules in the oral tissues, hence protecting the integrity of the gums and oral mucosa.

g. Tooth Support: While vitamin C primarily affects gum health, it indirectly benefits overall tooth health by improving the health of supporting structures such as gums and connective tissues.

h. Bone Health: The importance of vitamin C in collagen synthesis extends to bone health, which includes the jawbone, which supports teeth. The density of the jawbone is vital for tooth stability.

i. Wound Healing after Dental Treatments: Vitamin C's role in wound healing is important following dental treatments such as extractions or implants. Adequate vitamin C levels promote healing and lower the likelihood of problems.

j. Maintaining Saliva Production: Adequate hydration and vitamin C intake can help sustain saliva production, which is crucial for preventing dry mouth and supporting dental health.

Maintaining a balanced diet rich in vitamin C-rich foods, practicing excellent oral hygiene (brushing, flossing, and frequent dental check-ups), and quitting smoking are all significant steps toward better tooth health. If you have specific dental issues or conditions, speaking with a dentist or other oral healthcare specialist can offer you individualized advice targeted to your oral health needs.

Implications of Health and Deficiency

Due to its critical functions in several physiological processes, vitamin C deficiency can have serious health consequences. While severe vitamin C insufficiency is uncommon in modern countries, low vitamin C levels can still cause health problems. The following are some of the health consequences of vitamin C deficiency:

1. Scurvy: Severe vitamin C deficiency can result in scurvy, a disorder marked by weariness, weakness, swollen and bleeding gums, joint discomfort, anemia,

and skin problems. Scurvy, if not properly treated, can be fatal.

2. Impaired Collagen Synthesis: Vitamin C is required for collagen synthesis and a lack of it can lead to weakened connective tissues. Symptoms may include easy bruising, sluggish wound healing, and joint pain.

3. Gum Issues: Vitamin C deficiency can contribute to gum issues such as gingivitis and more severe gum disease (periodontitis). Symptoms include swollen gums and bleeding.

4. Skin Issues: Inadequate collagen synthesis and weaker skin structures can cause skin problems such as dryness, roughness, and sluggish wound healing.

5. Anemia: Vitamin C improves non-heme iron absorption from plant-based meals. Iron deficiency can result in decreased iron absorption and contribute to anemia.

6. Weariness and Weakness: Due to its function in energy metabolism and overall cellular health, vitamin C deficiency can cause weariness, weakness, and decreased energy levels.

7. Increased Infection Risk: Vitamin C helps the immune system, and a lack can impair

immunological function, making you more susceptible to infections.

8. Joint Pain: Due to its role in collagen formation, which is necessary for maintaining joint structures, deficiency may contribute to joint pain and discomfort.

9. Impaired Wound Healing: Vitamin C is required for normal wound healing, and a lack can result in slow and impaired wound and injury healing.

10.   Bone Health: Vitamin C deficiency can have an influence on bone health due to its function in collagen formation, which is necessary for bone strength and integrity.

11.   Cognitive Performance: While the exact mechanism is unknown, some evidence suggests that vitamin C insufficiency may be linked to cognitive impairment and decreased cognitive performance.

It's crucial to realize that even mild deficiency or low vitamin C levels can have health consequences, even if they're not as severe as full-blown scurvy. Maintaining a balanced diet rich in vitamin C-rich foods is critical for preventing deficiency. Citrus fruits, berries, kiwis, peppers, broccoli, and leafy greens are all high in vitamin C. If you suspect a vitamin C deficiency or have specific health concerns, see a doctor for a proper diagnosis and advice on how to address your dietary needs.

The Historical Significance of Scurvy

Scurvy is a medical illness caused by a significant lack of vitamin C, often known as ascorbic acid. Vitamin C is a necessary ingredient for the body's physiological functions such as collagen formation, wound healing, and antioxidant defense. Without enough vitamin C, the body's connective tissues, blood vessels, and skin become weakened, resulting in a variety of symptoms.

Scurvy symptoms can range in intensity and may include:

- Weakness due to fatigue
- Gums that are swollen and bleeding
- Joint discomfort
- Anemia
- Skin issues
- Wound healing takes time

Scurvy's Historical Context

Scurvy is a disease induced by a vitamin C deficit in the diet. It has long been an issue, particularly for sailors and explorers who started on long voyages without access to fresh fruits and vegetables.

Scurvy has a long history, dating back centuries, with documented examples dating back to ancient Egypt. However, the disease spread and became more prevalent throughout the Age of Discovery and Exploration, which lasted from the 15th to the 18th centuries.

Long sea expeditions were performed by European explorers during this period aboard ships that lacked sufficient storage facilities for fresh food. The sailors' diets were mostly made up of preserved, non-perishable goods such as salted meat, dried grains, and hard biscuits. The crews suffered from severe vitamin C insufficiency due to a lack of fresh fruits and vegetables, which are important sources of vitamin C.

Scurvy was widespread among sailors and had disastrous consequences for the health and well-being of nautical operations. If left untreated, symptoms included weariness, weakness, swollen and bleeding gums, joint discomfort, and, eventually, death.

Throughout history, different explorers and medics noticed the incidence of scurvy. The link between scurvy and food, notably a lack of fresh fruits and vegetables, was not identified until the 18th century.

James Lind, a Scottish naval surgeon of the Royal Navy, was a key figure in the fight against scurvy. Lind conducted trials on sailors suffering from scurvy in 1747 to investigate the efficacy of various therapies. His findings revealed that citrus fruits like lemons and oranges could be used to cure and prevent scurvy.

Although Lind's observations were regarded with suspicion at first, they soon gained acceptance, leading to the implementation of dietary adjustments onboard ships. The British Royal Navy, for instance, began distributing lemon or lime juice to sailors as a scurvy prevention method. This method dramatically reduced the disease's occurrence.

Over time, our understanding of scurvy and the necessity of vitamin C grew. The identification and isolation of vitamin C as the specific nutrient-preventing scurvy in the early twentieth century led to more effective therapies and prevention efforts.

Scurvy is now very uncommon in industrialized countries, mainly to improved dietary choices and year-round access to fresh fruits and vegetables. It can, however, occur in people who have limited access to varied and healthy food or who have specific medical disorders that interfere with vitamin C metabolism.

RDAs (Recommended Daily Allowances) for Vitamin C

The RDAs for vitamin C, also known as ascorbic acid, differ depending on age, gender, and stage of life. RDAs are established by health authorities to provide guidelines on the daily intake of nutrients required to meet the nutritional needs of the majority of people. The following are RDAs for vitamin C:

- Infants (from birth to 12 months):

  40 mg per day for children aged 0 to 6 months

  50 mg every day for 7 to 12 months

- Children:

  aged 1 to 3: 15 mg per day

  aged 4 to 8: 25 mg per day

aged 9 to 13: 45 mg per day

- Adults and Adolescents:

  Males aged 14 to 18: 75 mg per day

  Females aged 14 to 18: 65 mg per day

  Males aged 19 and up: 90 mg per day

  Females aged 19 and up: 75 mg per day

- Pregnant and Breastfeeding females:

  Pregnant females aged 14 to 18: 80 mg per day

  Breastfeeding females aged 14 to 18: 115 mg per day

  Pregnant women aged 19 and up: 85 mg per day

  Breastfeeding females aged 19 and up: 120 mg per day

- Smokers: Due to the increased oxidative stress induced by smoking, smokers should ingest an additional 35 mg of vitamin C each day.

It is crucial to note that these RDAs are only guidelines and may differ depending on individual health conditions, lifestyle circumstances, and unique requirements. Individuals who are pregnant or lactating, for example, may have increased requirements due to the demands of pregnancy and lactation.

Because vitamin C is water-soluble, it is not kept in the body for long periods of time and is expelled in the urine in excess. Consuming vitamin C-rich foods like citrus fruits, berries, kiwi, peppers, and leafy greens can help you achieve your daily vitamin C requirements. If you have special health issues, dietary limitations, or are contemplating vitamin C supplementation, you should seek personalized advice from a healthcare expert.

Current Research and Controversies Beyond the Common Cold

Vitamin C's importance goes beyond its relationship with the common cold, and continuous study is being conducted to investigate its potential benefits for a variety of health disorders as well as the controversy surrounding its use.

Here are some current vitamin C study areas and controversies:

1. Immune Support and Infections: While vitamin C is commonly connected with immune support, studies are being conducted to investigate its possible involvement in strengthening immune responses against infections other than the typical cold. Vitamin

C supplementation is being studied to see if it will help reduce the intensity and duration of respiratory illnesses such as influenza and pneumonia.

2. Antioxidant Effects: The antioxidant properties of vitamin C are being examined in relation to its ability to combat oxidative stress and inflammation. Research is being conducted to determine how these effects may lead to a reduction in the risk of chronic diseases such as cardiovascular disease and some types of cancer.

3. Cardiovascular Health: The effect of vitamin C on cardiovascular health is still being researched and debated. Some research suggests that consuming more vitamin C may be related to a lower risk of heart disease, whereas others have not consistently demonstrated such benefits. The role of vitamin C supplementation in reducing heart disease is still debated.

4. Cancer Prevention: Research on vitamin C's possible significance in cancer prevention is ongoing. According to some research, vitamin C's antioxidant qualities may help protect cells from DNA damage and aid the immune system's capacity to target cancer cells. However, the findings have been varied, and

additional research is required to establish a conclusive correlation.

5. Megadose Controversy: The assumption that high-dose vitamin C supplementation (megadose) can prevent or treat a variety of ailments, including cancer, has aroused debate. While some research has investigated high-dose vitamin C as an additional therapy, the evidence for its widespread use in mega doses for disease prevention is still lacking.

6. Wound Healing and Skin Health: Because of vitamin C's function in collagen formation, there has been increased attention to its potential advantages for wound healing and skin health. Vitamin C supplementation is being studied to see if it will improve wound healing and contribute to healthier skin.

7. Athletic Performance and Recovery: Some research has been conducted to determine whether vitamin C supplementation can increase athletic performance and minimize exercise-induced oxidative stress. The findings have been varied, with some research indicating possible benefits for specific populations.

8. Effect on Bone Health: The involvement of vitamin C in collagen synthesis has consequences for bone

health. The link between vitamin C intake and bone mineral density, fracture risk, and overall skeletal health is being studied.

9. Cognitive Function and Mental Health: New research is looking into the effects of vitamin C on cognitive function and mental health. Antioxidant effects and involvement in neurotransmitter production point to plausible connections, but additional research is needed to completely grasp these links.

As vitamin C research continues, it's crucial to remember that while some possible benefits have been revealed, not all studies are conclusive. A balanced diet rich in fruits and vegetables is the best source of vitamin C. If you're thinking about taking vitamin C supplements, especially at higher levels, talk to a doctor first to make sure they're right for you and that they're safe for your specific health needs and conditions.

Potential Side Effects of Mega dosing

Mega dosing is the practice of ingesting exceptionally high dosages of a certain substance, most commonly vitamins or minerals. While some may consider mega dosing as a means to gain optimal health advantages, it is crucial to realize that it might also result in significant adverse effects. These side effects differ based on the chemical being mega dosed, however here are a few examples:

1. Vitamin Toxicity: Excessive intake of some vitamins, such as A and D, can cause toxicity. Nausea, vomiting, headache, dizziness, exhaustion, hair loss, and even organ damage are possible symptoms.
2. Imbalances and Interactions: Excessive intake of certain vitamins or minerals might upset the body's nutrient balance. Excessive vitamin C intake, for example, may interfere with copper absorption and raise the risk of iron overload in persons with hemochromatosis.
3. Gastrointestinal Problems: Excessive amounts of some nutrients, particularly those obtained through supplements, can irritate the gastrointestinal tract, resulting in symptoms such as stomach cramps, diarrhea, and digestive difficulties.
4. Allergic Reactions: Some people are hypersensitive or allergic to specific substances. Mega dosing raises the risk of allergic responses, which can range from moderate skin rashes to severe anaphylactic shock.

5. Drug Interactions: Excessive dosage of certain substances might interfere with prescriptions a person is taking, potentially lowering their effectiveness or producing dangerous side effects. Before beginning any high-dose regimen, it is critical to consult with a healthcare expert.

6. Increased Tissue Damage Risk: Certain chemicals, such as fat-soluble vitamins, can accumulate in the body and cause tissue damage if ingested in extremely high concentrations over time.

7. Financial Costs: Mega dosing can be costly because high-dose supplements are frequently more expensive than regular-strength supplements. This expensive burden may not be worth the possible benefits, especially given the paucity of scientific data in favor of mega-dosing.

It is critical to underline that mega dosing should not be attempted without the supervision of a healthcare expert. A balanced and varied diet, supplemented, if necessary, as prescribed by a healthcare practitioner, is the best method to ensure optimal nutrient consumption.

The Benefits of Vitamin C

Vitamin C, commonly known as ascorbic acid, is a necessary nutrient with multiple functions in the body. Here are some of the potential advantages of vitamin C:

1. Antioxidant Activity: Vitamin C is a potent antioxidant that protects cells from free radical damage. This antioxidant activity may help to reduce the risk of chronic diseases like cardiovascular disease and certain types of cancer.
2. Immune System Support: Vitamin C is well-known for its involvement in immune function support. It promotes the formation of white blood cells, which are essential for combating infections. Adequate vitamin C levels can also improve immune cell activity and aid speedier wound healing.
3. Collagen Formation: Vitamin C is required for collagen production, a protein that gives structure to the skin, bones, tendons, and blood vessels. Sufficient consumption of vitamin C promotes healthy skin, wound healing, and general tissue restoration.
4. Iron Absorption: Vitamin C improves non-heme iron absorption, which is frequent in plant-based meals. Consuming vitamin C-rich foods or supplements alongside iron-rich meals might assist improve iron

status, particularly in people at risk of iron deficiency, such as vegetarians and women who have heavy menstrual bleeding.

5. Eye Health: Free radical oxidative stress and damage can lead to the development of age-related eye diseases such as cataracts and macular degeneration. The antioxidant effects of vitamin C may help minimize the risk of certain disorders and maintain healthy vision.

6. Heart Health: Vitamin C has been linked to a lower risk of cardiovascular disease. It may aid in the reduction of blood pressure, the improvement of blood vessel function, and the reduction of inflammation, all of which are significant elements in maintaining a healthy cardiovascular system.

7. Skin Health: Vitamin C is essential for the formation of collagen, which helps to preserve the skin's firmness and flexibility. Adequate vitamin C intake may aid in the reduction of age symptoms, wound healing, and overall skin health.

8. Stress Reduction: Vitamin C has been demonstrated to help reduce stress and improve mood. It participates in the synthesis of neurotransmitters such as serotonin, which govern mood and emotions.

It should be noted that, while vitamin C has potential benefits, excessive ingestion through mega dosing is not advised. The RDA for vitamin C varies by age and gender, and it is typically recommended to receive vitamin C through whole foods such as citrus fruits, strawberries, bell peppers, and broccoli rather than relying only on supplements. Before making any significant changes to your diet or supplementing routine, please consult with a healthcare practitioner.

CHAPTER FOUR: INTERACTION AND SYNERGIES

Interaction between Vitamin D and Vitamin C

Both vitamin D and vitamin C are essential nutrients with specific roles in the body, and they can interact in a variety of ways to benefit overall health. While these two vitamins have distinct activities, there are some interactions and potential synergy between them. The following is how vitamin D and vitamin C interact:

1. Immune Support: Both vitamin D and vitamin C perform functions in immune system support. Vitamin D regulates immunological responses and improves immune cell function, whereas vitamin C promotes immune cell activity and functions as an antioxidant to protect immune cells from oxidative stress. Adequate levels of these vitamins are required for a healthy immune system.

2. Anti-Inflammatory qualities: Vitamin D and C both have anti-inflammatory qualities. Vitamin D aids in the regulation of inflammation and immunological

responses, whilst vitamin C's antioxidant properties aid in the reduction of oxidative stress and inflammation in the body. Balanced amounts of these vitamins can help to improve the inflammatory response.

3. Collagen Synthesis and Skin Health: Vitamin C is required for collagen synthesis, which is necessary for skin health, wound healing, and connective tissue formation. Vitamin D is also important for skin health and cell differentiation. Adequate levels of these vitamins can help with skin health and wound healing.

4. Bone Health: Vitamin D is essential for bone health because it improves calcium absorption and promotes bone mineralization. The involvement of vitamin C in collagen formation is critical for bone structure. They work together to improve overall bone health.

5. Cardiovascular Health: Vitamin D and Vitamin C have both been related to cardiovascular health. Vitamin D helps the heart by regulating blood pressure, lowering inflammation, and increasing endothelial function. The antioxidant properties of vitamin C aid in cardiovascular protection. A healthy

balance of both vitamins may have a synergistic effect on heart health.

6. Mood Management and Cognitive Health: Vitamin D is involved in mood management and cognitive function, while the antioxidant qualities of vitamin C improve brain health. Maintaining adequate levels of these vitamins has the potential to improve mental health.

7. Improved Nutrient Absorption: Some research suggests that vitamin C may improve nutrient absorption, particularly non-heme iron and maybe vitamin D. More research, however, is required to completely comprehend these connections.

8. Anti-Infection Benefits: Vitamin D and vitamin C have both been studied for their ability to lower the severity and duration of respiratory infections. While vitamin D helps antimicrobial peptides in the respiratory tract, vitamin C's immune-boosting qualities can aid in the fight against infections.

9. Oxidative Stress Reduction: The anti-inflammatory properties of vitamin D can indirectly help to reduce oxidative stress. They can help protect cells from oxidative damage when paired with vitamin C's direct antioxidant effects.

While there are interactions between vitamin D and vitamin C, they are separate nutrients with different roles. A balanced diet rich in vitamin D and vitamin C sources, such as fatty fish, fortified foods, citrus fruits, berries, and vegetables, is the best way to maintain optimal levels of both vitamins. If you're thinking about taking supplements, go to a doctor first to evaluate your specific needs and make sure you're not exceeding safe intake amounts.

Effects of Combination on Immune Function

Because both vitamins play important roles in supporting many parts of the immune system, the combined impact of vitamin D and vitamin C on immunological function can be significant. While their mechanisms of action are diverse, their synergistic contributions can result in better immune responses and overall immunological health. The following is how vitamin D and vitamin C work together to support immunological function:

1. Immune Cell Regulation: Vitamin D aids in the regulation of immune cells such as T cells and macrophages. It helps to balance immunological responses by encouraging the development of

regulatory T cells, which serve to prevent excessive inflammation. Vitamin C also promotes immune cell activity and assists immune cells in performing at their best by shielding them from oxidative stress.

2. Antioxidant Protection: Both vitamin D and vitamin C have antioxidant characteristics that aid in the neutralization of free radicals and the reduction of oxidative stress. They help to maintain the integrity and activity of immune cells, allowing them to respond effectively to infections by minimizing oxidative damage.

3. Antimicrobial Peptide Production: Vitamin D stimulates the production of antimicrobial peptides like cathelicidin and defensins, which are part of the body's natural defense against infections. These peptides aid in the direct combat of pathogens as well as the regulation of immune responses. The immuno-supportive characteristics of vitamin C supplement these acts by enhancing total immune cell function.

4. Improved Barrier Function: Vitamin D helps to maintain the integrity of epithelial barriers such as the skin and respiratory lining. This barrier is important in keeping infections from entering the body. The significance of vitamin C in collagen

production promotes the health and integrity of these barriers.

5. Immunological System Coordination: Both vitamin D and vitamin C help to coordinate immunological responses. Vitamin D helps the immune system respond correctly to diverse types of threats, whereas vitamin C helps immune cells communicate and signal.

6. Lower Infection Risk: Adequate amounts of vitamin D and vitamin C help reduce the risk of infections, particularly respiratory infections. The significance of vitamin D in increasing innate immunity, as well as the immuno-modulating and antioxidant effects of vitamin C, create a favorable environment for the immune system to successfully combat infections.

7. Immune System Resilience: The combined actions of vitamin D and vitamin C can help to make the immune system more resilient. They aid the immune system in responding quickly to infections, reducing inflammation, and protecting immune cells from harm.

8. Overall Health and Wellness: A healthy immune system is essential for overall health and wellness. Both vitamin D and vitamin C promote good health

by supporting several physiological activities other than immune responses.

9. Individual Variation: It is crucial to highlight that individual characteristics such as genetics, lifestyle, and underlying health issues can all have an impact on how vitamin D and vitamin C interact in the context of immune function. Consultation with a healthcare practitioner can assist in determining the optimal intake of these vitamins based on individual needs.

Consuming a well-balanced diet rich in vitamin D and vitamin C, getting enough sun exposure for vitamin D synthesis, and considering supplementation, when necessary, can all help to improve immune function and overall health. If you're thinking about taking supplements, talk to a doctor about the best dose for you based on your specific health situation.

Skin Health Potential Synergies

When it comes to skin health, vitamin D and vitamin C may have synergistic effects. Both vitamins serve unique but complementary functions in skin health, and their combined activities can improve skin function, appearance, and overall well-being. Here's how vitamin D and vitamin C complement each other to promote skin health:

1. Collagen Synthesis and Skin Structure: Vitamin C is required for collagen synthesis, a process that gives the skin structural support. Collagen aids in the maintenance of skin elasticity, firmness, and durability. Vitamin D promotes skin cell proliferation and differentiation, which helps to produce healthy skin layers.

2. Wound Healing: The role of vitamin C in collagen formation is critical for wound healing. Collagen serves as a scaffold for tissue repair, whereas vitamin D promotes the immune response and skin cell regeneration required for effective wound healing.

3. Antioxidant Protection: Both vitamins have antioxidant characteristics that protect skin cells from oxidative stress produced by UV rays, pollution, and other environmental factors. Vitamin C directly neutralizes free radicals, but vitamin D contributes to antioxidant protection indirectly by improving the skin's inherent defense systems.

4. Skin Barrier Function: Vitamin D aids in the maintenance of the skin's barrier function. This

barrier protects the skin from dangerous bacteria and avoids excessive moisture loss. The role of vitamin C in collagen production aids in the creation of a robust and effective skin barrier.

5. UV Protection: While vitamin D is created in reaction to sunshine, excessive UV exposure can cause skin damage. The antioxidant properties of vitamin C serve to combat UV-induced oxidative stress and reduce the risk of solar damage. Both vitamins' combined effects help to protect the skin from UV radiation.

6. Skin Aging: Factors related to skin aging include collagen breakdown, oxidative stress, and decreased skin cell turnover. These concerns are addressed by both vitamin D and vitamin C. Vitamin C increases collagen synthesis and reduces oxidative damage, whilst vitamin D promotes cell regeneration and aids in the maintenance of skin health over time.

7. Inflammatory Skin problems: The anti-inflammatory actions of vitamin D can help those with inflammatory skin problems such as acne, psoriasis, and eczema. The antioxidant and anti-inflammatory effects of vitamin C help to soothe and improve these illnesses.

8. Skin Brightening and Even Tone: Because vitamin C inhibits melanin formation, it can help to improve skin tone and minimize hyperpigmentation. Vitamin D helps to maintain a healthy complexion by supporting the skin's natural coloring.

9. Skin Hydration: Both vitamins help to keep the skin hydrated. Vitamin C promotes the formation of hyaluronic acid, which aids in the retention of moisture in the skin. Hydration is critical for plump, healthy-looking skin.

10. Overall Skin Wellness: The combined actions of vitamin D and vitamin C enhance overall skin wellness by supporting structural integrity, environmental stressor protection, and the ability to repair and regenerate.

To take advantage of the possible synergy between vitamin D and vitamin C for skin health, eat a well-balanced diet high in vitamin D and vitamin C sources including fatty fish, citrus fruits, berries, and vegetables. Furthermore, sun safety, such as minimizing UV exposure and applying sunscreen, is critical for protecting the skin while allowing for appropriate vitamin D production. If you're thinking about using these vitamins in skincare or supplements, go to a dermatologist or healthcare professional for specific advice.

Considerations for Enhancement

When contemplating vitamin D and vitamin C supplements, there are several crucial variables to consider to ensure that you're making informed and safe decisions. Here are some important considerations:

1. Individual Requirements: Determine whether you have a special supplements requirement. Before beginning any supplementing routine, contact a healthcare expert to evaluate whether you have a vitamin deficit or inadequate intake of these vitamins.
2. Dietary Consumption: Examine your current vitamin D and vitamin C intake. It is generally preferable to receive nutrients from a well-balanced diet rich in whole foods. Supplementation may be recommended if your diet lacks sufficient sources of these vitamins.
3. Dosage Recommendations: Understand the recommended dietary allowances (RDAs) for vitamin D and vitamin C. Age, gender, health state, and life stage can all influence the optimal dosage. Without

professional advice, do not exceed the suggested dosages.

4. Vitamin D Source: Sunlight, food sources, and supplementation are all sources of vitamin D. If you're thinking about taking a vitamin D supplement, talk to your doctor about whether you should take vitamin D2 or vitamin D3, as the two have different effects on blood levels.

5. Formulations and Combinations: Think about the supplementing form - capsules, tablets, liquids, or gummies. Vitamin D may also be combined with vitamin C or other elements in some supplements. Choose formulations that are compatible with your preferences and any dietary constraints.

6. Medication Interactions: Check to see if any of your drugs interact with vitamin D and vitamin C pills. These vitamins may interact with certain drugs, such as steroids or anticoagulants.

7. Health Concerns: Before beginning any supplementing plan, speak with your healthcare physician if you have any underlying health concerns, are pregnant, or are breastfeeding. Your healthcare professional can give you advice that is suited to your individual health needs.

8. Monitoring and Testing: If you choose to supplement, consider having your blood levels checked on a regular basis to verify you are not exceeding safe levels and to track the impact of supplementation on your health.

9. Balance and Variety: Supplements should supplement, not replace, a healthy lifestyle and balanced diet. Using supplements only while ignoring dietary and lifestyle aspects may not produce the best outcomes.

10. Quality and Brands: Select reputable brands and goods that have been quality tested and meet industry requirements. On the supplement label, look for third-party verification markings.

11. Potential Side Effects: Be cautious of the risks associated with excessive doses of these vitamins, particularly mega dosing. Excessive vitamin D intake, for example, can cause toxicity and other health problems.

12. Long-Term Approach: Think about supplementing as part of a long-term health strategy. Reassess your nutritional needs on a regular basis and speak with a healthcare expert if your circumstances change.

Remember that, while supplements can be beneficial for individuals with deficiencies or specific needs, the cornerstone of good health is a well-balanced diet and lifestyle. Consultation with a licensed dietitian, nutritionist, or healthcare expert can assist you in making informed supplementing decisions based on your unique health objectives and circumstances.

CHAPTER FIVE: PRACTICAL TIPS FOR BALANCED VITAMIN INTAKE

The Importance of a Well-Balanced Diet

A well-balanced diet is necessary for good health and well-being. It gives the body the perfect balance of nutrition, energy, and vital components it needs to function and grow. Here are some of the main reasons why a well-balanced diet is essential:

1. Nutrient Intake: A well-balanced diet provides a variety of critical nutrients such as vitamins, minerals, carbs, proteins, fats, and fiber. Each vitamin serves a unique purpose in the body, and deficiencies or excesses can cause health problems.

2. Energy Supply: The body requires energy to accomplish basic processes like breathing as well as more complicated operations like exercise and cognitive function. A well-balanced diet delivers the energy needed to meet these demands from a variety of sources.

3. Development and Growth: Proper nutrition is critical for growth and development, particularly in children and adolescents. Proteins, vitamins, and minerals aid in the creation of tissues, bones, and organs.

4. Weight Management: By supplying the proper quantity of calories and nutrients, a balanced diet will help you maintain a healthy weight. A proper balance of carbs, proteins, and lipids promotes metabolic health and lowers the risk of obesity.

5. Disease Prevention: A diet high in fruits and vegetables, whole grains, lean proteins, and healthy fats has been linked to a lower risk of chronic diseases like heart disease, diabetes, and some types of cancer.

6. Digestive Wellness: A fiber-rich diet promotes digestive health by reducing constipation, facilitating regular bowel movements, and supporting gut-bacteria balance.

7. Immune Function: Nutrient-rich foods, such as those high in vitamins A, C, D, and zinc, assist the body fight against infections and illnesses.

8. Cardiovascular Health: A balanced diet high in fiber and low in saturated and trans fats promotes cardiovascular health by maintaining good

cholesterol levels, blood pressure, and general heart function.

9. Cognitive Function: Nutrients such as omega-3 fatty acids, antioxidants, and vitamins contribute to brain health, cognitive function, and the prevention of neurodegenerative illnesses.

10. Mood and Mental Health: Nutrient shortages can have an impact on mood and mental health. A nutrient-dense diet promotes neurotransmitter synthesis, which is necessary for emotional well-being.

11. Bone Health: Adequate calcium, vitamin D, and other mineral intake promotes bone health and lowers the risk of osteoporosis.

12. Skin Health: Vitamins C and E, as well as antioxidants, contribute to skin health by promoting a young appearance and guarding against UV damage.

13. Longevity and Quality of Life: Eating a well-balanced diet has been related to living a longer and healthier life. It improves general vitality, energy levels, and the ability to fully enjoy life.

Remember that a balanced diet is more than simply particular items; it is also about the entire eating routine. A balanced diet emphasizes moderation, diversity, and portion control. It is advised to eat whole, minimally processed meals and to seek individualized advice from healthcare specialists or registered dietitians based on your specific nutritional needs and health goals.

Meal Planning and Dietary Sources

A well-balanced diet entails including a variety of nutrient-rich foods in your meals and snacks. To assist you in achieving optimal nutrition, below is a guide to food sources and meal planning:

1. Vegetables and Fruits: Vegetables and fruits are rich in minerals, fiber, vitamins, and antioxidants. Incorporate varieties of vegetables and fruits into your meal. Leafy greens, berries, citrus fruits, carrots, broccoli, and bell peppers are among the examples.
2. Whole Grains: Whole grains contain a variety of complex carbohydrates, fiber, vitamins, and minerals. For long-lasting energy, choose whole wheat, brown rice, quinoa, oats, and whole grain bread.
3. Lean Proteins: Include poultry, fish, eggs, tofu, legumes (beans, lentils, chickpeas), and low-fat dairy products as lean protein sources. These give amino acids that are required for tissue repair and growth.

4. Healthy Fats: Include avocados, nuts, seeds, olive oil, and fatty fish (such as salmon and mackerel) in your diet. These fats promote heart health, brain function, and fat-soluble vitamin absorption.

5. Dairy or Dairy Alternatives: Select low-fat or non-fat dairy products, as well as fortified dairy alternatives such as almond milk, soy milk, or yogurt. These contain calcium, vitamin D, and protein, all of which are beneficial to bone health.

6. Portion Management: To avoid overeating, pay attention to portion proportions. A serving of protein is around the size of your palm, a serving of grains is about the size of your cupped hand, and a serving of fats is about the size of your thumb.

7. Meal Preparation: Plan meals that include a variety of macronutrients (carbohydrates, proteins, and fats) as well as micronutrients (vitamins and minerals). To achieve your nutritional requirements, include a range of food types.

8. Hydration: Drink plenty of water throughout the day. Water is required for digestion, vitamin absorption, and other biological activities.

9. Snacking: Snack on nutrient-dense foods such as fruits, vegetables, nuts, yogurt, and whole grain

crackers. These can assist to normalize blood sugar levels and keep you from overeating at big meals.

10.   Conscious Eating: Train yourself to be conscious of your hunger and fullness signs. Slow down and savor your food's flavors, textures, and colors.

11.   Limit Processed Foods: Limit your intake of highly processed foods, which are frequently heavy in added sugars, harmful fats, and sodium. When possible, use whole, minimally processed foods.

12.   Variety: Change up your dietary selections to ensure you're getting a variety of nutrients. Experiment with new recipes and cuisines to keep your meals fresh.

13.   Special Dietary Needs: If you have certain dietary restrictions, allergies, or medical issues, consult a qualified dietitian to develop a meal plan that matches your individual requirements.

14.   Balanced Meals: Include a source of lean protein, complex carbohydrates, healthy fats, and lots of veggies in your meals. This combination delivers long-term energy as well as adequate food intake.

Remember that eating a healthy diet is a long-term commitment to your overall health. Small modifications made over time can lead to long-term improvements.

Meal planning, frequent physical activity, and consultation with healthcare specialists or licensed dietitians can all aid in the achievement and maintenance of nutritional goals.

When and How to Use Supplements

Supplements can help fill dietary shortfalls and support specific health needs. However, they must be used with caution and under the supervision of healthcare professionals. When and how to use supplements efficiently are outlined below:

1. Determine Your Nutritional Needs: Before you consider supplements, determine your dietary intake and potential nutrient shortages. A certified dietician or healthcare physician can assist you in determining which nutrients you may require supplementation.

2. Medical Conditions: Certain medical conditions or health situations may need the use of supplements. Consult your healthcare professional to evaluate whether supplements are required depending on your specific health profile.

3. Nutrient Testing: If you feel you have a nutrient shortage, consider getting a blood test to check your

nutrient levels. This will help determine whether and how much supplementation is required.

4. Quality is Important: Select reputable brands that conform to quality and safety regulations. On supplement bottles, look for third-party testing and verification labeling.

5. Dosage: Follow the dosage recommendations on the supplement label or as directed by your healthcare provider. More is not necessarily better; excessive consumption might have negative consequences.

6. Food First: When feasible, prioritize obtaining nutrients from entire foods. Supplements should not be used in place of a well-balanced diet, but rather to supplement it.

7. Individual Needs: Supplement requirements differ from person to person. What works for one individual might not work for another. Avoid imitating someone else's supplement routine.

8. Seek Professional Advice: Before beginning any supplements, speak with a qualified dietitian, nutritionist, or healthcare provider. They can give you specific advice based on your medical history and needs.

9. Interactions: Be careful of any potential interactions between your supplements and drugs. Certain pairings can have negative consequences.

10. Focused supplementing: Consider focused supplementing for certain situations such as pregnancy, breastfeeding, or established deficits.

11. Duration: Supplements may be required for a short period of time to repair a deficiency or to support a specific health goal. Long-term use should be guided by periodic evaluation and professional advice.

12. Avoid Mega dosing: Avoid mega dosing on supplements because excessive intake can result in negative side effects, toxicity, and imbalances.

13. Monitor Effects: Keep track of how supplements influence your body. If you notice any side effects or reactions, stop using it immediately and consult a medical professional.

14. Periodic Re-evaluation: Review your supplement program on a regular basis. Nutrient requirements can alter over time, so it's critical to modify your supplements properly.

Remember that supplements should never be used in place of a well-balanced diet and an active lifestyle. Aim to receive nutrients largely from whole meals while selectively using supplements to suit specific needs. It is critical to consult with a healthcare practitioner to ensure that you are using supplements safely and efficiently.

Professionals in Healthcare Consultation

Speaking with a healthcare professional before making supplementing decisions is critical to ensuring that you're making informed and safe choices for your health. Here's why and how you should seek medical advice:

Why Seek the Advice of Healthcare Professionals?

1. Personalized Advice: Doctors, licensed dietitians, and nutritionists, for example, can make individualized suggestions based on your specific health status, medical history, and needs.
2. Accurate Evaluations: They can determine whether you have any nutrient deficits or health issues that may necessitate supplements. Blood testing and medical evaluations can provide useful information.
3. Potential Interactions: Healthcare providers can assess the possibility of interactions between supplements and prescriptions you are taking. Some

supplements can reduce the effectiveness of some medications or aggravate pre-existing disorders.

4. Appropriate Dosages: They can assist in determining the proper dosage of supplements to avoid overdoing them, which could result in negative effects.

5. Evidence-Based Information: Healthcare providers can provide evidence-based information regarding the advantages and hazards of supplementing, allowing you to make more educated decisions.

How to Speak with Healthcare Professionals

1. Make an Appointment: Make an appointment with your primary care physician, a registered dietitian, or a nutrition-focused healthcare specialist.

2. Prepare yourself: Gather information about your current food, lifestyle, medications, and any symptoms you may be having before the meeting.

3. Pose a Question: Do not be afraid to ask questions during the appointment. Discuss your worries, the reasons you're thinking about taking supplements, and any current health conditions.

4. Share Additions: Inform your doctor about any supplements you are already using. Bring the supplement labels or an ingredient list to your consultation.

5. Follow Suggestions: Your healthcare practitioner will provide suggestions based on your talk. This could offer specific supplements, doses, and safe-use advice.

6. Regular Check-Ins: If you are prescribed supplements, your healthcare physician will most likely urge periodic check-ins to monitor their effectiveness and, if necessary, change the regimen.

Additional Suggestions

- Keep Up to Date: Learn everything you can about the supplements you're thinking about buying. Look for trustworthy sources of information and be wary of falsehoods.

- Take a Look at the Big Picture: When providing suggestions, healthcare professionals examine your general health, medical history, and lifestyle. They'll make sure supplements are part of a well-rounded health strategy.

- Don't Rely on the Internet Alone: While online resources can be useful, they should not be used in place of expert advice. Incomplete or incorrect information can exist. It is important to note that what works for one person might not work for another. Recommendations should be tailored to your individual needs.

- Stay away from self-diagnosis and self-treatment: Self-diagnosis of deficiencies or health issues, as well as self-prescription of supplements, can be dangerous. Allow experts to influence your decisions.

Remember that your healthcare practitioner is a partner in your health. Their knowledge will assist you in making decisions based on your specific needs, ensuring that you are on a safe and successful route to well-being.

Vitamin Intake Monitoring and Adjustment

It is critical to monitor and adapt your vitamin intake to ensure that you are getting your nutritional needs without exceeding safe amounts. Here's a strategy to efficiently monitor and adjust your vitamin intake:

1. Routine Health Exams: Make an appointment with your primary care physician or healthcare professional on a regular basis. They can run blood tests to check your nutrient levels and discover any deficits.

2. Speak with a Registered Dietitian: A trained dietician can assist you in developing a balanced meal plan that matches your individual nutritional requirements. They can advise you on proper food choices and, if necessary, supplementation.

3. Keep a Food Journal: Track your daily food intake to keep track of your nutrient intake. There are numerous apps and online programs that can assist you in keeping track of your meals and nutrient intake.

4. Recognize Dietary Sources: Learn about foods that are high in the vitamins you're worried about. This will allow you to make more educated decisions and ensure variety in your diet.

5. Adhere to Dietary Guidelines: Adhere to national dietary guidelines that prescribe daily vitamin intake. These recommendations are frequently dependent on age, gender, and life stage.

6. Keep an Eye on the Symptoms: Take note of any symptoms that may indicate a deficit. Fatigue, weakness, brittle nails, and skin changes, for example, could be symptoms of vitamin deficiencies.

7. Adjust for Special Circumstances: Your vitamin intake may need to be adjusted in certain scenarios.

Pregnancy, nursing, illness, stress, and increased physical activity are all examples of conditions in which your vitamin requirements may increase.

8. Use Supplements Wisely: If you use supplements, do it under the supervision of a healthcare expert. Unless otherwise instructed by a physician, do not exceed the specified dose.

9. Regular Blood testing: Get regular blood testing to check your vitamin levels. Based on your health situation, your healthcare professional can recommend the proper frequency for these tests.

10. Seek Professional Advice: Consult a healthcare physician or trained dietician if you are concerned about your vitamin consumption or suspect a deficit. They can make suggestions for changes to your diet or supplement routine.

11. Be Wary of Excess: While it is critical to achieve your vitamin requirements, overdoing it can be harmful. Certain vitamins, such as fat-soluble vitamins (A, D, E, and K), can build up in the body and cause toxicity.

12. Pay Attention to Your Body: Your body frequently sends forth messages regarding its nutritional requirements. Cravings for particular

foods may indicate a deficit. However, consulting with professionals is still necessary before making major adjustments.

13.	Balanced Diet Approach: Make a balanced diet rich in whole foods a priority. Supplements may not deliver the same benefits as acquiring nutrients from a variety of food sources.

Keep in mind that vitamin consumption is only one part of your total health. Consultation with healthcare professionals will assist you in making informed decisions about modifying your vitamin consumption based on your specific needs.

CONCLUSION

For this reason, vitamins are often referred to as the "building blocks" of good health. These important nutrients serve a critical part in a variety of biological activities, ranging from energy production to immune system strength. Understanding and prioritizing the importance of vitamins in overall health is essential for living a bright and balanced life.

The Basis for Vital Processes: Vitamins operate as coenzymes, assisting enzymes in carrying out critical chemical processes that keep our bodies running smoothly. Vitamins are necessary for every metabolic action, from transforming food into energy to aiding the creation of critical chemicals.

Resilience of the Immune System: Certain vitamins, such as vitamin C and vitamin D, are essential for boosting our immunological defenses. Vitamin C is a powerful antioxidant that fights free radicals and supports immune cells. Vitamin D aids in the regulation of immunological responses and improves the body's ability to fight infections.

Cellular Maintenance and Repair: Vitamins are required for the proper maintenance and repair of our cells and tissues. They aid in the creation of collagen, the protein that serves as the foundation for skin, blood vessels, bones, and other structures. Adequate vitamin consumption guarantees that our bodies can repair and regenerate effectively.

Vitamins operate as defenders against oxidative stress, a process that can harm cells and contribute to chronic diseases. Antioxidant vitamins, such as vitamin C and vitamin E, help to prevent cellular damage by neutralizing free radicals. B vitamins, such as B6, B12, and folate, are essential for maintaining a healthy neurological system. They help to produce neurotransmitters, which regulate emotion, cognition, and overall brain function.

A Comprehensive Strategy: While vitamins are unquestionably important, they are only one component of the picture. Physical activity, stress management, sleep, and mental well-being are all components of a holistic approach to health. Vitamins work in tandem with these elements to form a solid foundation for overall health.

Personalization and Knowledge: Each person's vitamin requirements vary depending on characteristics such as age, gender, health issues, and lifestyle. This underlines the significance of making educated decisions. Making sound selections requires consulting with healthcare specialists and being up to date on reputable dietary information.

Recognizing and understanding the critical role of vitamins in general health is the first step toward creating a robust and thriving body and mind in an era where wellness is a priority.

Finally, vitamins D and C are vital nutrients that play critical roles in overall health and well-being. Their roles in the body are diverse, ranging from bone health and immunological function to wound healing and antioxidant protection. As previously discussed, vitamin D is known as the "sunshine vitamin" due to its production from sunlight, whereas vitamin C is well-known for its antioxidant effects and crucial involvement in collagen synthesis.

These vitamins are important not only for individual health but also for public health initiatives and illness prevention. Adequate vitamin D and C intake are critical for promoting optimal health throughout the lifespan. While getting these vitamins from whole foods is best, supplementing under the supervision of a healthcare practitioner can help address deficits or special health needs.

Staying educated is critical in an era of individualized nutrition, technology developments, and growing research. Consultation with healthcare specialists, measuring your nutrient consumption, and adapting your food and lifestyle to the most recent scientific findings can enable you to make informed decisions regarding your vitamin D and C intake. Remember that vitamins are only one part of a comprehensive approach to health that includes eating a balanced diet, keeping active, managing stress, and getting enough sleep.

Your dedication to knowing and harnessing the power of vitamins D and C will add to your general well-being and vitality as the landscape of health and nutrition evolves.